Ellie Herman's
Pilates
Props Workbook

Ellie Herman's

Pilates
Props Workbook

Step-by-step guide
with over 350 photos

photography by Robert Holmes

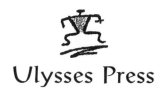

Ulysses Press

Published in the United States by
Ulysses Press
P.O. Box 3440
Berkeley, CA 94703
www.ulyssespress.com

ISBN10: 1-56975-414-4
ISBN13: 978-1-56975-414-6
Library of Congress Control Number 2004101021

Printed in Canada by Webcom

10 9 8 7 6 5 4 3

Editorial/Production	Lily Chou, Claire Chun, Steven Zah Schwartz, James Meetze, Samantha Glorioso
Indexer	Sayre Van Young
Design	Sarah Levin
Photography	Robert Holmes
Models	Anya Schmidt, Carie Lee, Caleb Rhodes, Susan Volkan, Ellie Herman, Cathryn Yost

Distributed iby Publishers Group West

Please Note
This book has been written and published strictly for informational purposes, and in no way
should be used as a substitute for consultation with health care professionals. You should not
consider educational material herein to be the practice of medicine or to replace consultation
with a physician or other medical practitioner. The author and publisher are providing you
with information in this work so that you can have the knowledge and can choose, at your
own risk, to act on that knowledge. The author and publisher also urge all readers to be
aware of their health status and to consult health care professionals before beginning any
health program.

contents

part one:

getting started

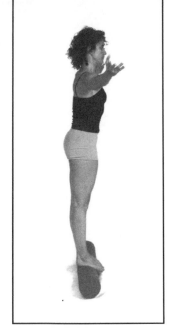

introduction

My torrid romance with Pilates began many years ago when I was a professional dancer and choreographer with my own dance company in San Francisco. To supplement my paltry income and to satisfy my desire for edgy experience, I decided to try my hand as a professional wrestler. My career as "Ruth Less" was cut short by a serious knee injury, which occurred during a tag-team match.

At the time I cursed myself for being so stupid: How could I have taken my body for granted, especially being a dancer. I thought for sure my life as a dancer was over.

But then I learned about St. Francis Hospital DanceMedicine in San Francisco, where I ventured to heal myself with this mysterious thing called Pilates. I was lucky enough to be put under the care of Elizabeth Larkham, one of the superstars of modern Pilates.

After months of Pilates rehabilitation and no surgery (normally advisable after an anterior cruciate ligament tear), I returned to dancing only to realize that, to my surprise, I was a much better dancer than before my injury. Pilates had not only allowed me to return to

jumping, leaping, and twirling, it had actually improved my technique, control, balance, and core strength. At this moment, I became a Pilates convert.

I then moved to New York City, where I briefly attended the Masters program in dance at New York University. The best thing about my short stay at NYU was the morning Pilates mat class with Kathy Grant, one of the disciples of Joe Pilates. She taught me how depth and creativity could be brought to the Pilates method, while getting me out of the mounting hip pain that was due to the ballet classes I was taking every day. These Pilates classes inspired me to pursue Pilates teacher training with Romana Kyranowska, another of Joe Pilates original students.

I returned to San Francisco in 1992 and continued my study of Pilates with Jennifer Stacey and Carol Appel of Body Kinetics. The following year I opened my own studio in my live/work loft in the Mission district of San Francisco. The studio expanded so much over the years that we moved to a bigger building, with two full floors dedicated to Pilates-based fitness, rehabilitation, teacher training, continuing education, and complementary medicine. As the demand for good Pilates instruction grew, so did my business, and I opened a second studio in Oakland, California, in 2001. Somewhere during all this expansion I managed to earn a Master of Science degree in Acupuncture & Chinese Herbal Medicine.

HOW PROPS SAVED MY LIFE

After my knee injury, I thought for sure I would never dance again. I was humbled by my disability, unable at first to even walk, and later full of fear that I would re-injure myself. But then a wonderful doctor gave me a Thera-Band exercise band and told me how to use it. He gave me two simple exercises; the hamstring strengthener (essential for an anterior cruciate ligament tear) and the quad strengthener. I went home, sat on my chair, and did those darn exercises, no matter how boring. And lo and behold, my knee felt immediately more stable. Later, I did some fancier rehabilitation on the Pilates equipment, but what got me back on my feet was the elastic exercise band. I am forever indebted to that thin ribbon of rubber!

I've now taught Pilates for over ten years and have developed a unique language with which to communicate the essence of the Pilates method. Please see the section entitled Ellie Herman's Pilates Alphabet for my particular Pilates terms and concepts, used throughout the book. I hope these tools help you to understand the subtleties of Pilates in both a physical and conceptual way.

As part of my ongoing interest in Pilates innovation, I have developed a new piece of Pilates equipment called the Pilates Springboard, an inexpensive and space-saving variation of the Wall Unit/Cadillac. You can find out more about the Pilates Springboard on my website www.ellie.net, where you can also find information on my other upcoming projects, including a video you can use with this book.

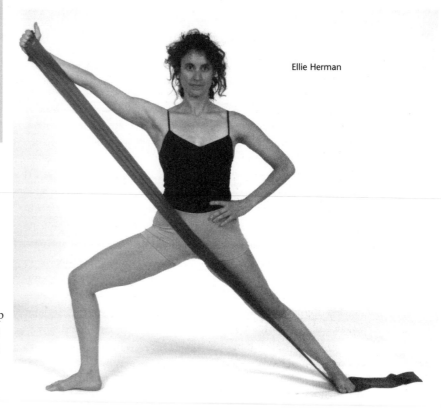

Ellie Herman

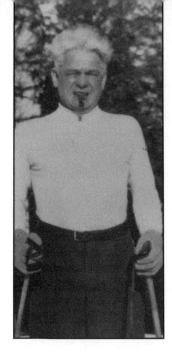

the story of Joe

The story goes that Joseph Hubertus Pilates was born in Germany in 1880, and as a child suffered from asthma and a sunken chest. He spent his life obsessed with restoring his health and body condition. Over his lifetime, he overcame his frailties and became an accomplished athlete. He loved skiing, diving, gymnastics, yoga, and boxing. There are famous pictures of the man looking extremely fit well into his 70s—doing Pilates exercises in the snow.

Originally Joe developed a series of mat exercises designed to build abdominal strength and body control. He then built various pieces of equipment to enhance the results of his expanding repertoire of exercises. His idea behind building the equipment was to replace himself as a spotter for his clients.

How He Invented the Pilates Equipment

Stationed in an English internment camp during WWI, Pilates rigged springs above hospital beds, allowing patients to rehabilitate while lying on their backs. This particular set-up later evolved into the Cadillac, one of the main pieces of Pilates equipment. He then developed over 20 contraptions—some of which look a little like medieval torture devices—constructed of wood and metal piping, using a variable combination of pulleys, straps, bars, boxes, and springs.

In his words, the Pilates method "develops the body uniformly, corrects wrong postures, restores physical vitality, invigorates the mind, and elevates the spirit." Joe was way ahead of his time, viewing the body holistically and emphasizing the body working as a whole unit.

Through the decades, Pilates developed over 500 exercises, which he originally called Contrology, but have since come to be known as the Pilates method.

In 1923 Joseph Pilates emigrated to the United States, settling in New York City, where he opened a studio on Eighth Avenue in Manhattan and started training and rehabilitating professional dancers (George Balanchine and Martha Graham were two of his students).

Joe's Legacy

The original Eighth Avenue Pilates studio in Manhattan is where the first generation of teachers were trained, including Romana Kyranowska, Kathy

Grant, Ron Fletcher, Eve Gentry, Carola Trier, Mary Bowen, and Bruce King. These protégés branched out and opened studios around the country, changing the method based on their own individual backgrounds and philosophies. For the following 50 years or so, the Pilates method has been passed down through many more generations of teachers and has transformed a great deal along the way. Some of the New York teachers claim to hold truest to the "original" method, but many creative individuals have brought their own insights to improve upon some of the more antiquated views of the body. Joe was a trailblazer, but his ideas can be improved upon. Even within his lifetime, he evolved his repertoire and changed his approach to better attain his desired results.

Pilates Now

Today, the Pilates method consists of a repertoire of over 500 exercises to be done on a mat or on one of the many pieces of equipment Joseph Pilates invented. The exercises are usually done in a series organized by levels: beginning, intermediate, advanced, and super-advanced. Pilates exercises as a whole develop strong abdominal, back, butt, and deep postural muscles to support the skeletal system and act as what Pilates called the "powerhouse" of the body. The Pilates method works to strengthen the center, lengthen the spine, increase body awareness, build muscle tone, and gain flexibility. The Pilates method is also an excellent rehabilitation system for back, knee, hip, shoulder, and repetitive stress injuries. Pilates addresses the body as a whole, correcting the body's asymmetries and chronic weaknesses to prevent re-injury and bring the body back into balance. As Joe used to say, "after 10 sessions you'll notice a difference, after 20 sessions other people will notice a difference, after 30 sessions you'll have a whole new body."

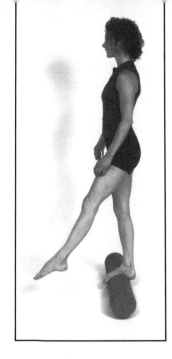

how to use this book

This book is filled with a wide variety of exercises. Some are classic Pilates mat exercises using a prop. Others are specific exercises for rehabilitation or special problems. Please see the Suggested Workouts section on page 29 for ideas on how to put together a workout if that's what you seek, or how to approach a specific injury or issue that ails you.

The Levels

Do the beginning exercises until you feel comfortable with the concepts and the movements. Then add the intermediate exercises. After a few months of conditioning, you can try the advanced and super-advanced exercises.

Remember, the levels of the exercises are meant to help you learn the Pilates method in a natural progression for your body. Most importantly, the levels are meant to help you not hurt yourself. The intermediate and advanced exercises require a fair amount of core strength to perform properly. You could injure your back if you try to push yourself beyond your level.

Please read the Dos and Don'ts for each exercise carefully to make sure you are performing the exercise with the correct form. If you feel strain in your low back or neck at anytime, please do not continue with the movement, but look for modifications instead.

When learning new exercises, it is common for certain aches and pains to develop. The following are a few common problems that people face when they are still in the process of

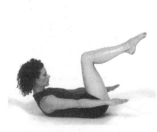

Protect your low back: 1 Beginning

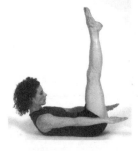

2 Intermediate

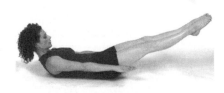

3 Advanced

gaining strength and stability. Please read through this section even if you don't have any of these problems yet. The point is to prevent potential overuse or strain of your muscles and tissues.

How to Modify to Protect Your Low Back

In general, if you suffer from low back pain, you need to know a few tips to keep you from further contributing to your problems. Always modify any exercise that requires you to support your legs out in front of you while keeping your belly scooped or your back flat on the mat. Experiment with the following modifications:

- Bend your knees if the exercise requires straight legs.
- Keep your legs high enough so that you can absolutely maintain a scooped belly and a flat back on the mat.
- Stop if you feel back strain.

How to Avoid Wrist Compression When Up on Your Arms

- Spread your fingers and press into all of them when weight-bearing. Focus especially on pressing into the thumb, forefinger, and pinky.
- Try to "cup" your wrist when weight-bearing. That is, lift up the middle of your palm to decrease putting weight into your wrist joint proper.
- Keep your shoulders properly aligned. Think of rolling the shoulder blades down away

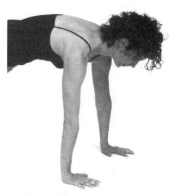

Correct: Lift up from the wrists and shoulders and soften the elbows.

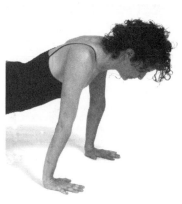

Incorrect: Avoid dropping into your wrists, elbows, and shoulders.

from the ears so you are supporting your body weight with the back muscles.
- Think of pressing away from the ground with your back strength.
- Don't let your weight bear down into the wrist; instead, press away from gravity.
- Don't hyperextend your elbows: keep the inner elbow creases facing each other.

How to Do a Rolling Exercise: Never onto Your Neck!

There are several exercises on the floor in which you are required to roll onto your upper back (Rolling Like a Ball, Open Leg Rocker, Rollover, etc.).
- Do not roll onto your neck; instead, stop and balance between your shoulder blades.
- Use control when rolling back. Don't roll back so fast that you can't control your momentum.
- Scoop your abdominals in to help stop yourself from rolling back too far.
- You should be able to lift your head off the mat as a test to see if you've rolled back too far.

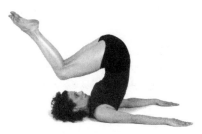

Incorrect neck placement: Don't roll onto your neck.

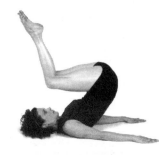

Correct neck placement: Balance between your shoulder blades.

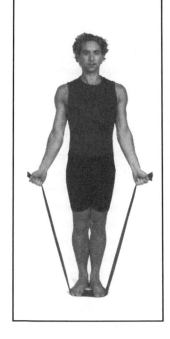

eight principles of Pilates

Joseph Pilates' book, *Return to Life*, maps out the eight important principles that underlie the Pilates method. When Pilates exercises are done with the following concepts in mind, you will gain much more depth and effectiveness in your workout.

Control

As I mentioned earlier, Joseph Pilates originally called his method "Contrology" (it wasn't until his students began teaching for him that people started referring to the method as Pilates). One of the fundamental rules when doing Pilates: Control your body's every movement! This rule applies not only to the exercises themselves but also to transitions between exercises, how you get on and off the equipment, and your overall attention to detail while working out. When doing mat exercises, control comes into play with the attack and ending of each movement. When the body puts on the brakes in a controlled manner, it is training the muscles to work as they lengthen. This is called eccentric muscle contrac-

tion, which builds long and flexible muscles. Also, when focusing on control of a movement, the body is forced to recruit helper muscles (we call these synergists), which are usually smaller than the main muscles. When many muscles work together to do one movement, or when muscles work synergistically, the body as a whole develops greater balance and coordination. Also, the big muscles won't get too big and bulky because they don't have to do all the work by themselves. Thus we become a long and lean machine. Once your body learns to move with control, you will feel more confident doing all kinds of things from hiking a rocky cliff, to salsa dancing, or to standing on a chair to reach an out-of-the-way martini glass.

Breath

I have heard that most people use 50 percent of their lung capacity when they breathe. Shallow breathing is an unfortunate side effect of a sedentary and stressful life. Moreover, people actually hold their breath when performing a new or difficult task. When training Pilates clients, I have to tell them to exhale or else often they won't! When you hold your breath, you tense muscles that can ultimately exacerbate improper posture and reinforce tension habits. That is why consistent breathing is essential to flowing movement and proper muscle balance. As with yoga, breathing is an essential part of the Pilates method and distinguishes it from other exercise forms.

Every Pilates exercise has a specific breathing pattern assigned to it. Breathing while moving is not always an easy assignment, but when accomplished, beautiful things can happen. Focused breath can help maximize the body's ability to stretch, and through this release of tension you will gain optimal body control. Deep inhalation and full exhalation also exercises the lungs and increases lung capacity, bringing deep relaxation as a pleasant side effect.

Flowing Movement

Many of the moves in Pilates look a lot like yoga. But unlike yoga, we do not hold positions—instead we flow from movement to movement. In this way Pilates is more like dance, in that the flow of the body is essential to doing Pilates correctly. When doing a Pilates workout, you want to flow and move freely during the movement phase and finish with control and precision. This way of moving brings flexibility to the joints and muscles while training the body to elongate and move with an even rhythm. Flowing movement integrates the nervous system, the muscles, and the joints, and trains the body to move smoothly and evenly.

Precision

Precision is a lot like control but has the added element of spatial awareness. When attacking any movement you must know exactly where that movement starts and ends. All Pilates exercises have precise definitions of where the body should be at all times: the angle of the legs, the placement of the elbows, the positioning of the head and neck, even what the fingers are doing! The little things count in Pilates. This kind of precision in movement will resonate in the rest of your life. If you suffer from pain because of faulty postural habits that you aren't even aware of, after a few good sessions with a competent Pilates instructor, you will be pleasantly surprised by how fast a new-found awareness can affect a positive change in your body. This change can only happen when you begin to notice your physical habits and increase the precision in your movements.

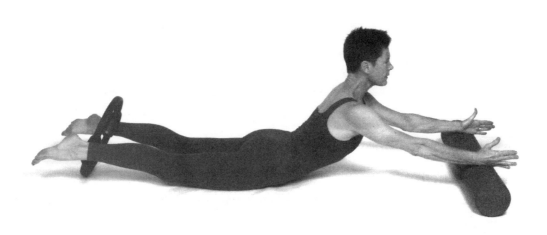

Centering

Sometimes we joke at my studio that we should have subliminal tapes running all day that say "Pull the navel to the spine." Why? Because this is the mantra of any worthy Pilates trainer. All exercises are done with the deep abdominals engaged to ensure proper centering. Most Pilates exercises focus on developing abdominal strength either directly or indirectly. Never forget to pull in the belly or you will be reprimanded by the Pilates Goddess! Even when performing an exercise that focuses on strengthening the arm muscles, you should keep your abdominal scoop, keep your shoulders pulling down the back, and perhaps even squeeze your butt. All these actions promote centering and core muscle strength. No exercise should be done to the detriment of center control. In other words, if your center is not totally and completely engaged and stabilized, you may not progress to the next level of an exercise.

Stability

Ever wonder what makes Pilates such an excellent back rehabilitation method? The lion's share of Pilates exercises utilize the concept of torso stability, which is key to the health and longevity of your spine. Now what is stability? Basically, it is the ability to not move a part of the body while another part is challenging it. Maintaining stillness in the spine as you move the arms and legs requires torso stability, accomplished mainly by the abdominal muscles. After an injury, there is generally instability in the affected area. The first thing you want to do is learn to stabilize the injured part so as to prevent re-injury and to allow the healing process to begin. Thus, Pilates is one of the safest forms of exercise to do after injury. Pilates will also prevent injury, for if you have excellent stability in your torso and joints, you are much less likely to injure yourself in the first place.

Range of Motion

"Range of motion" is a phrase used by medical professionals to describe how much movement a part of the body can perform. For instance, the range of motion of your shoulder joint is defined by how high you can raise your arm in front of you, behind you, etc. Your range of motion can be affected by your muscles, bones, and other tissues such as ligaments and fascia (connective tissue). Basically, range of motion is just another way of describing flexibility. Pilates exercises are meant to increase the range of motion of your spine or joints if you are too tight. If you are too flexible (yes, this is possible!), Pilates exercises will help you to learn the proper range of motion for your spine or joints. It is important to understand how to limit your range of motion if you lack stability because this will help to prevent injury in the future.

Opposition

In any great story there is a protagonist and an antagonist, the hero and the bad guy. Similarly, for each muscle in your body there is an opposing muscle that performs an opposite movement. These are called agonists and antagonists. If the agonist is tight, the antagonist will be weak or will be unable to contract fully. This is an essential concept to grasp when conditioning your body. If you wonder why it's so hard for you to straighten your legs in front of you when sitting up, it's because your hamstrings are tight. Your quadriceps are the muscles that straighten your legs, but if your hamstrings are super-tight, then the quads have to work overtime to straighten the legs.

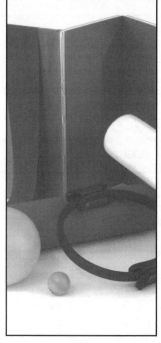

Pilates and props

If variety is the spice of life, then props would be the salt on your Pilates mat, enhancing the flavor and effect of Pilates matwork. In some cases, a prop makes an exercise more difficult, creating a stability challenge or increasing the work on one part of your body (e.g., the magic circle between your ankles transforms the Hundred, a classic torso stability exercise, into a terrific inner thigh exercise, and also adds some weight to the legs, which increases the stability challenge).

In other cases, a prop makes an exercise easier (e.g., in the Open Leg Rocker, putting your feet in the magic circle instead of holding the legs with your hands allows those with tight hamstrings greater ease in extending the legs).

Some of the exercises are not Pilates at all, but classic rehabilitation exercises aimed at specific body parts (e.g., the exercise band Shoulder Series). The magic circle and the towel, in fact, are the only classic Pilates props. The other props in the book—the roller, elastic exercise band, and the pinkie ball—are more modern additions to my Pilates repertoire. We use these props at my studio because sometimes it's simply the best way to target a specific problem (for instance, the roller Basic Shoulder Set is hands down the best way to release and open the chest, align the neck and shoulder, and alleviate upper back and neck pain). Read on for specifics about each prop.

Elastic Exercise Bands

Exercise bands have been used by physical therapists for years to aid in rehabilitation, and allow patients to do home programs. In this book, I transform classic Pilates mat and equipment exercises to incorporate these elastic bands. Adding resistance to an exercise can sometimes make the exercise more difficult for the targeted muscle group, or can make the exercise easier by assisting you in completing a movement.

These bands come in different colors that denote different resistances. The Thera-Band company, one of the more popular makers of the prop, uses a color-coded progressive resistance system. In order from lightest to heaviest: yellow, red, green, blue, black. Other companies use different colors, so you must research each company's system to make sure the resistance is right for you. Most of the exercises in this book were done with a blue Thera-Band, or a "medium heavy" one.

You can also buy handles to put on the ends of the exercise band to aid in proper alignment and provide comfort when holding the ends with your hands. Also, you can buy an accessory that allows you to easily attach the band to a door knob for your rehab exercises.

General Rules: Never strain yourself. Instead, use a lighter "weight" until you can perform the exercise with ease. If you are injured, start with a lighter weight and progress upward. That's the whole point of this progressive resistance concept—it allows you to gain strength at your own pace. Don't be macho with rehab!

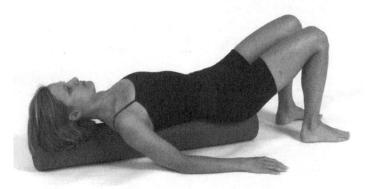

Ethafoam roller

Use the following guidelines to help you choose the correct weight for your exercises.

- *Knee strengthening:* heavy to extra heavy
- *Shoulder strengthening:* light to medium
- *Full-body mat exercises:* heavy

Roller

The roller is sometimes called the Feldenkreis roller after Moishe Feldenkreis, a brilliant body worker who developed a system called "Awareness through Movement," or just "Feldenkreis"; he used the roller in some of his exercises. The roller is made of ethafoam, a styrofoam-like material that can get flattened over time, especially if you stand on it; it's sold by packing and shipping companies as well as many therapeutic and fitness distributors. Everyone in my studio loves the roller once they've tried it; there is something really comforting about lying down on a white log and releasing the tensions of the day. People automatically feel the benefits, particularly of

the Basic Shoulder Set that I lay out in the beginning of the roller section. The roller is one of the best-selling props in my studio.

Like the exercise band, the roller is used by physical therapists, but for different reasons. The roller is an unstable surface upon which you must learn to stabilize, thus making basic mat exercises much more challenging. If you find an exercise too challenging on the roller, one basic modification is just to do it on the floor first, then add the roller when you're able.

Pinkie Ball

Yes, it's the same ball that you played handball with as a child.

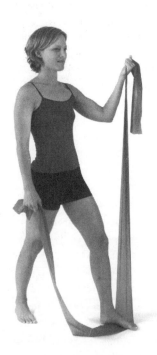

Elastic exercise band

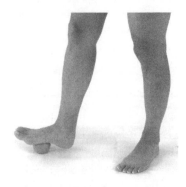

Pinkie ball

Just think, now you can re-experience your childhood while releasing all that adult tension you've been building up all these years. The pinkie ball is used in my studios for muscle and fascial release.

Towel

Okay, so there's only one towel exercise, but it's good and classic Pilates. Try it if you have flat feet or weak arches.

Magic Circle

According to Pilates lore, Joseph Pilates used to enjoy drinking beer at his studio on Eighth Avenue in New York and would order kegs to be delivered regularly. Being the crazy genius that

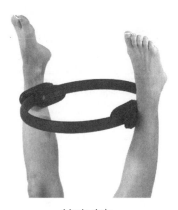

Magic circle

he was, one day he removed the ring from the keg and put wooden blocks on either end. This was the birth of the "magic circle" (it must have seemed magical after a keg of beer!). So don't complain if you think the pads on your circle aren't cush enough; just think back to the

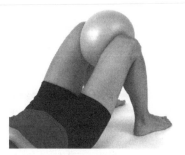

In many exercises, a child's play ball can be substituted for the magic circle.

wooden blocks and be happy that we have kinder, gentler manufacturers than Joe.

If you don't want to invest $30–$60 in a circle, you can do many of the exercises with a child's play ball, given that it's somewhat squishy and rebounds when you squeeze it. Overball and Gertie Ball make great balls to hold between your ankles and knees. I still think the circle is better than a ball in most cases just because it's more intense and has a direct line of resistance—you can only squeeze it in one direction. The ball has a gentler resistance and is softer to hold, so it's nice if you have an injury or feel that the circle is too heavy for you to support.

For the most part, the magic circle is a great way to really work your inner and outer thighs on many Pilates mat exercises.

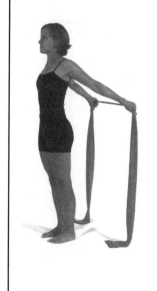

general movement vocabulary

Articulation

This is another word for range of motion. We use this word mainly when referring to moving the spine one vertebra at a time while rounding down the mat, as opposed to coming down in one piece.

Extension

Technically, extension is a movement that brings a part of the body backward from its normal anatomical position, but we also use extension to mean *to straighten*—as in "straighten your knee." It can also mean *to lengthen* or *stretch*, as in "extend your arms and legs long on the mat." Extension of the spine is when the spine arches back, opening the belly, while the head or tail move backward or toward each other; the Swan movement is a perfect example of this principle.

Flexion

Flexion is the opposite of extension: it's a movement that brings a part of the body forward from its normal anatomical position. It also means *to bend*, as in "flex your knee." Flexion of the spine is the movement that brings the head forward (closer)

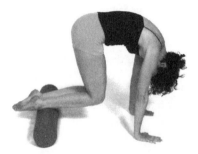

Flexion of the spine, shoulders, hips, and knees

to the pelvis or vice versa; the C-curve or any abdominal curving exercise is a good example of this.

Parallel vs. Turn-out

If you've ever taken a modern dance class, you've probably heard the terms parallel legs and turned-out legs. Simply put, parallel means your knees face forward, as most of us do naturally when we stand. Turn-out or external rotation of the hips means your knees and feet are facing away from each other and

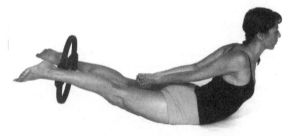

Extension of the spine, shoulders, hips, and knees

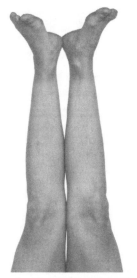

Turned-out legs; Pilates First Position

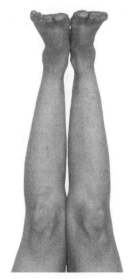

Parallel legs

your leg bones are laterally rotated in the hip socket. All ballet dance is done in turn-out, while modern dance often has movements that use the legs in parallel. In Pilates, we do many exercises in turn-out (see Pilates "V" from the Pilates Alphabet on page 25). Why turn-out? Because it engages both the butt and inner thighs, and can help stabilize your pelvis during certain exercises.

Supine

This is a term that simply means lying on your back. Think spine (supine with the "u" taken out).

Prone

This term means lying on your belly.

The Powerhouse

The Powerhouse is a term that came from Joe Pilates himself, used today mostly by New York trainers. The abdominals, butt, and inner thigh muscles, when working together, constitute the Powerhouse. This is where many of the Pilates exercises can be initiated. It is also the area that is challenged in many exercises. These muscles are the main stabilizing muscles of the body and are very important for preventing injury to the spine.

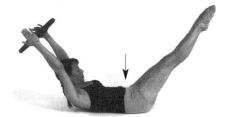

The Powerhouse

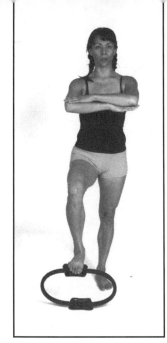

Ellie Herman's Pilates alphabet

Just as every word can be broken down into letters, so can every Pilates exercise be broken down into discrete parts. The Pilates alphabet is my way of facilitating the learning process and demystifying even the most complex Pilates exercises. Almost every advanced exercise contains basic movements that repeat over and over in the repertoire.

Abdominal Scoop

The Abdominal Scoop can be done anywhere and at any time, and frankly it should be done as much as possible. Pulling the navel in toward the spine, thinking of zipping up a tight pair of pants, or sucking in your spare tire will all do the job. What you are doing anatomically is engaging your deepest abdominal muscles, which function to hold in your viscera and, when con- tracted, decrease the diameter of the abdominal wall. The Abdominal Scoop works a lot like a drawstring around a pair of sweat pants when pulled taut. You have four layers of abdomi- nal muscles; your deepest one is called the *transversus abdominis*. The second and third layers are called your *internal* and *external obliques*. And the most superfi- cial abdominal layer is called your *rectus abdominis*. The rectus (as we Pilates instructors call it) is a workaholic muscle and will do all the work if you let it. The Abdominal Scoop, or "navel to spine" image is meant to bring in the deeper three layers, which work to compress the abdominal wall and help support the back. In every exercise you want to be using your Abdominal Scoop to get the most profound results possible. Pooching is the oppo- site of scooping—No pooching allowed!

Balance Point

Balance Point is a position in which you begin and end the rolling exercises in the Pilates mat repertoire; it is also the place you arrive at the top of the

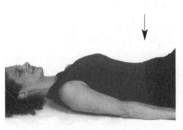

Here Susan is scooping.

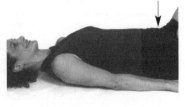

Here Susan is pooching:
No pooching allowed!

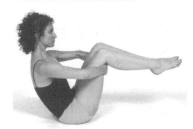

Balance point

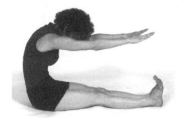

C-curve

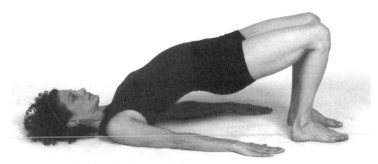

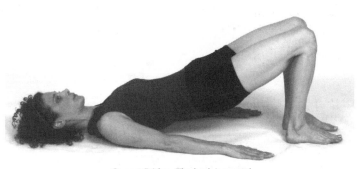

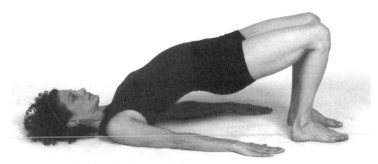

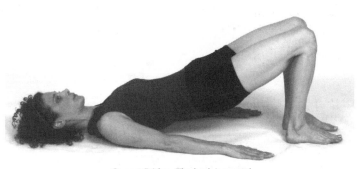

Teaser. You can practice Balance Point by sitting up with your knees bent, holding on to the backs of your thighs. Roll back slightly behind your tailbone, pull your belly in, and lift your feet off the floor. In order to maintain your balance and stop yourself from rolling backward, you must engage and pull in your deep abdominal muscles and slightly round the low back. This teaches you that to balance with ease, you must engage your deep abdominals.

Bridge

Bridge is a basic position in Pilates as well as a beginning-level exercise on the mat and the ball. In kinesiological terms, a Bridge is extension of the hips. In lay terms, this means lifting your hips up off the floor, using your butt and hamstrings to do so. It's part of the Pilates Alphabet because it is a position we come in and out of during various exercises. I want to point out that a Bridge should be done from the hip extensors (butt and hamstrings) and not from the back muscles. Therefore, when doing a Bridge, you must keep your spine neutral and make sure not to arch the back!

C-Curve

Martha Graham was the first person to introduce the idea of C-curve into modern dance. Before Graham, dancers performed ballet or used the Isadora Duncan technique, which has the spine always erect, extended, elegant, and otherworldly. Graham introduced spinal flexion, or what she termed "the contraction," which revolutionized dance. It was a primal, dark, and

oh-so-human movement. It put us back onto the earth from some other world. Joe Pilates worked with Graham in his Eighth Avenue studio and learned a couple of tricks from her. The C-curve is rounding of the back, or flexion of the spine. The "C" is meant to describe the shape of the back after you scoop in your belly. This shape should always be initiated by your deep Abdominal Scoop and should provide a lovely stretch for your spine. Many Pilates exercises use the C-curve.

Door Frame Arms

Arms are straight in front of you, shoulder distance apart, making the shape of the outer frame of a door. This describes the shape of your arms in many Pilates exercises, whether your arms are

Correct Bridge: The back is neutral.

Incorrect Bridge: The back is hyperextended.

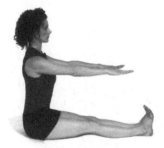

Door Frame Arms

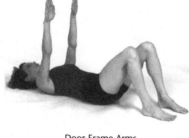

Door Frame Arms

above your head, by your sides when lying supine on the floor, or supporting you in a plank position.

Hip-up

The name says it all. Lie on your back with your legs up, your knees bent, and your Door Frame Arms down by your sides. Rock back and lift your hips up by using your low Abdominal Scoop. The Hip-up works your lower abdominals and can be very challenging for those with a weak tummy, a tight back, or a large butt!

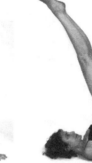

Hip-up

Levitation

When you combine a Hip-up with a little low butt squeeze, you get Levitation. What the low butt squeeze is actually doing is extending the hip. In kinesiolog-

ical terms, a Hip-up by itself is merely the flexion of the spine, but when you squeeze your butt, you add an extension of the hips—put them together and you have Levitation. Try it if you like: lie on your back, lift up your hips with your Abdominal Scoop, and at the top of the Hip-up, squeeze your butt. You'll feel your hips levitate, rising percep-tibly higher, as if the hand of Houdini came down and lifted your hips magically and effort-lessly off the floor.

Levitation

Neutral Spine

If you've ever wondered what the heck the difference is between the New York and the West Coast Pilates schools, I've

got two words for you: Neutral Spine. Neutral Spine is one of the most subtle yet powerful principles in Ellie Herman's Pilates Alphabet. Like much of Pilates, understanding Neutral Spine requires an understanding of your body and anatomy. Neutral Spine can be felt when lying down on your back, knees bent and feet flat on the floor. Your spine should have two areas that do not touch the floor beneath you: your neck and your low back (cervical and lumbar spine, respectively). One way to visualize Neutral Spine is to imagine you have a pitcher of hot water balanced on your low belly. When you are in neutral, your pitcher should not spill and should be perfectly balanced. If your pelvis is tilted forward (arching your low back too much off the floor) or tilted pos-teriorly (flattening your low back onto the floor), your pitcher will spill in one of those directions. Your tailbone should be grounded onto the floor.

To get technical: Neutral pelvis is actually defined as the pubic bone and the hip bones (*anterior superior iliac spine*, or the ASIS for short) being on the same plane. You can feel these bony landmarks with your fin-gers when you're lying down, and this triangle of bones, when neutral, should create a flat table for your pitcher. The reason we care about Neutral Spine is that this is the healthiest position for your spine when standing up—when your spine is neutral you have natural curves. These

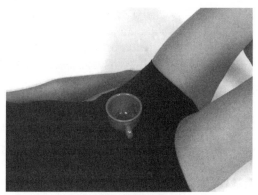

Correct Neutral Spine

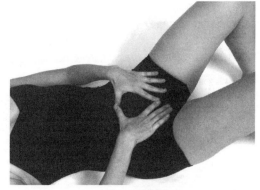

Defining Neutral

curves function to absorb shock when running, jumping, or simply walking around town. And ultimately if you live in Neutral Spine, you will be putting the least amount of stress on the muscles and bones. That's the beauty of perfect posture: it actually feels better. We want to maintain and reinforce these natural curves and that is why we often work in Neutral Spine when performing stability exercises in Pilates. Many people from the New York school teach people to "tuck under" or flatten the curve of their low back when doing Pilates exercises or when standing. This method is no longer thought to be posturally correct; instead, the natural curve or Neutral Spine is preferred.

Pilates Abdominal Positioning

The Pilates Abdominal Positioning is my way to describe the placement of the upper body when performing many of the supine Pilates floor exercises. When lying on your

back (supine), lift your head off the floor just high enough so that the bottom tips of your shoulder blades are either just touching or just off the floor. Imagine that the base of the sternum is anchored to the floor and the back of the neck and upper back are stretching around that anchor. Make sure to keep a space the size of a tangerine under your chin (see below); you are not meant to overstretch the back of your neck. It is essential to maintain this position when performing abdominal exercises. If you allow the head to drop back, you will begin to feel fatigue in the neck and you will not be using your abdominals as much. The upper

abdominals should be working to maintain this position (and that's where you should feel the burn).

Pilates "V" (Pilates First Position)

If you've ever taken a dance class, you probably know that First Position means standing with your legs together and turned out from the hip, knees facing away from each other, and feet making a V shape. The Pilates V is very much the same, except you never want to force the turn-out. Your feet should be making a V shape, but I always say this V should be the shape of a slice of pie, not a huge slice but a nice small Pilates-size slice.

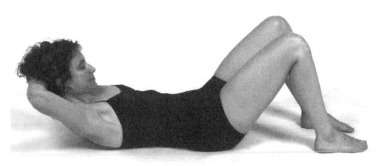

Pilates Abdominal Positioning

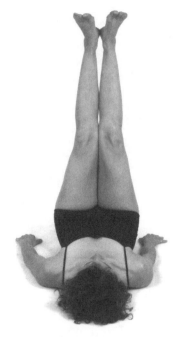

Pilates First Position

In Pilates, instead of keeping your legs parallel, we use this First Position in many exercises. Why? Because externally rotating the hips engages the gluteus maximus and the inner thigh muscles, which we like to use as much as possible in Pilates. (See Parallel vs. Turn-out, page 20.)

Rosebud

Have you ever gotten a bunch of roses and one of them has a broken bud? You know, one bud that droops down sadly, almost detached from its stem. If you imagine your head as the bud and your spine as the stem in a healthy unbroken rose, then in any movement your spine makes the bud will follow and continue the curve of the spine in a smooth line. When you move your head in a "faulty" sequence (say, when you come up into a

Swan or perform back extension from lying on your belly), your head can look like a broken bud; that is, your neck is bent at a greater angle than the rest of your spine. We want no broken buds in Pilates! Only healthy, happy roses and spines.

Squeeze a Tangerine

This is an image that describes the sequencing of your head as you lift it off the floor. It also shows the distance your chin should be from your chest when holding your Pilates Abdominal Positioning. The size of a tangerine is precisely the amount of space that should be between your chin and your chest when doing a spinal flexion.

Stacking the Spine

Stacking the Spine is a finish to several exercises in the Pilates method. Stacking the Spine teaches spinal articulation as well as how to sit up vertically.

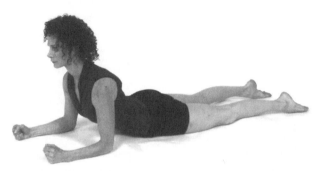

Correct neck placement: Rosebud atop stem

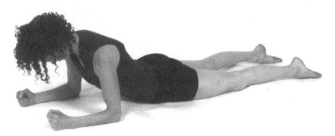

Broken Bud: Too much flexion

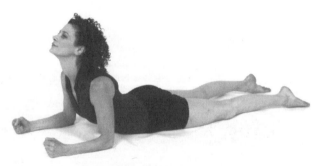

Broken Bud: Too much extension

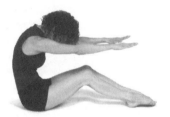

Stacking the Spine 1

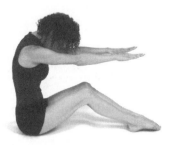

Stacking the Spine 2

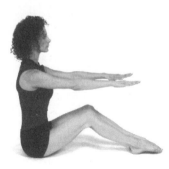

Stacking the Spine 3

It is a way to sit up or stand erect from a hunched-over position. Stacking the Spine begins with the lowest part of the spine and stacks up, one vertebra at a time, the head staying heavy and dropped until the very end. The spine should be completely vertical at the end, with the natural curves of the back in place. (This can be practiced against a wall to better feel the vertical alignment of the spine.)

Table Top Legs

Table Top Legs describes the position of your legs when you are lying supine (on your back), with the knees and feet up off the floor, inner thighs pulling together, knees bent at a 90-degree angle, and the thighs at a 90-degree angle to the floor.

Torso Stability

Torso stability is accomplished mainly by abdominal strength and is one of the most important concepts in the Pilates method. Most Pilates exercises require you to maintain a stable torso while the arms or legs move. Again, the abdominals are responsible for keeping the spine still while forces are moving around it. So when you are doing one of these stability exercises (and you can tell if it is a stability exercise if you hold the torso in one place for the duration of the exercise), simply think to yourself, "Don't move." This is the essence of stability.

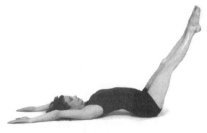

Poor Torso Stability:
Incorrect placement of the spine

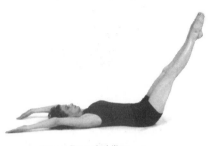

Strong Torso Stability:
Correct placement of the spine—abdominals keep the back flat on the floor

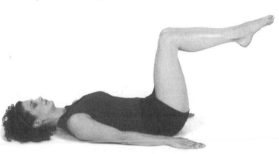

Table Top Legs

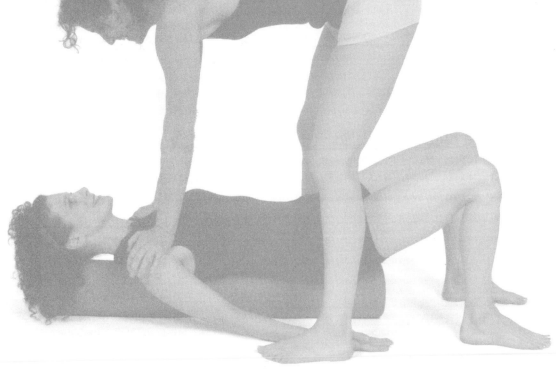

part two:

suggested workouts

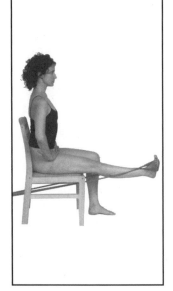

home programs

The props in this book are used by physical therapy patients to facilitate and accelerate rehabilitation. If you suffer from a strain, injury, or chronic problem, consult the following section on how to strengthen your weak areas. Remember to check with your physician or health-care professional before beginning any new exercise routine.

In this chapter you'll find programs that address injuries and painful conditions in the following areas:

- lower back
- shoulder
- knee
- neck and upper back tension
- ankle instability
- flat feet/fallen arches

Types of Injuries

Injuries have two very general categories:

1) **Acute injuries** are caused by an excessive force on a joint, muscle, tendon, or ligament. This may cause sudden onset of pain, swelling, fear of movement, and the sensation of instability (in the case of shoulder instability, the arm feels like it's hanging by a thread). Most acute injuries are caused by trauma that induces excessive movement in a joint (shoulder, knee, hip, wrist, spinal segment), which then results in instability in that joint. In order to heal and protect it from re-injury, we must regain the stability in the joint. Often, we need to become stronger than we were before the injury to ensure that no further damage will occur due to the instability.

2) **Chronic conditions** have many causes: some are internally degenerative processes such as arthritis, multiple sclerosis, or simple aging; others can be due to misalignment, microtraumas, or repetitive movements that over time damage the joint tissues. Chronic conditions tend to cause intermittent discomfort or pain that may get worse over time, and may be accompanied by weakness and decreased range of motion. Also, they can be caused by instability or joint laxity, which makes one more prone to injury. It can be very helpful to see a specialist when trying to rehabilitate a chronic problem since it is important to understand the underlying causes and rule out any potential serious diseases. When we have degenerative conditions, we must work with what we have. Carefully strengthen and regain as much range of motion and strength as possible.

Repetitive Strain

Our bodies were not meant to do micromovements. Nor were we designed to lift heavy objects day after day. When we have an injury due to repetitive strain, we must stop doing that movement. If our livelihood depends on it, we must try to find a way to perform the movement with the most efficiency and least strain on the injured area. If you work at a desk, see a specialist to make your work station ergonomic. If you do physical labor, be sure to learn proper body mechanics when bending and lifting. The most basic rule is to keep your spine neutral when bending forward and/or lifting something heavy. Never load the spine when it is rounded.

Inflammation

Inflammation is our body's way of telling us to lay off while it sends healing juices to an injured area. Thus, inflammation initially after a trauma is a good thing, but over time it stops the related joint/area from being able to heal properly and can be a hindrance to rehabilitation. I had a teacher once who described inflammation as a traffic jam, where everything gets congested and nothing can move through. Don't try to rehabilitate when you are still in the acute inflammation phase of an injury. Once the swelling has gone down, try to gingerly begin your home program. You may have to do a dance with inflammation; experiment with just how much you can do without causing yourself pain. Anti-inflammatories and ice in the beginning phases of rehabilitation and after exercise can be very helpful, but be judicious in your use of anti-inflammatories because recent research has shown that they may impede the healing of ligaments and tendons. It is normal

for inflammation to come and go when you are first rehabilitating an injury. Don't get dismayed if, say, your knee hurts a little after you complete your home program…ice it and keep your chin up.

The Psychology of Pain and Healing

From my experience, the rehab process is a rocky road, and it's important to keep up your spirits. Find a new hobby that doesn't involve the affected area. Post-injury is often a great time to reevaluate your life and try something new. Think of it as an opportunity, not just a problem. Research has shown that chronic painful conditions are best alleviated by heavy exercise…so don't be afraid to sweat a little! Babying yourself hasn't shown to be an effective way to get out of pain.

Principles of Rehabilitation

Here are the seven golden rules when it comes to rehabilitation:

- When we have tightness, we must stretch or release.
- When we have weakness, we must strengthen.
- When we have instability, we must stabilize.
- When we have misalignment, we must re-align.
- When we have a repetitive strain injury, we must stop doing that movement!

With these principles in mind, I've created two-part Home Programs that will facilitate a

quicker and more effective healing process. In order to correct imbalances we must 1) *stretch and release tight areas* then 2) *strengthen and stabilize weak and unstable areas.*

Phase 1: Stretch and Release Tight Areas

When it comes to releasing muscles on the pinkie ball or roller, the best way to know if you need a particular muscle release is to try the exercise, see if the muscle feels particularly tight or bound up (usually denoted by pain upon pressure), and see if you feel better afterward. You may feel immediate relief of your symptoms after releasing certain muscles, if they are the underlying cause of your problem. The same goes for the stretching exercises. You may not need to do all the release exercises mentioned in the programs. Basically, listen to your body!

Phase 2: Strengthen Weak Areas

In the following Home Programs you will have a list of strengthening exercises, all of which target certain areas. These are broken down into "Essential" exercises, as well as "Supplemental" moves to do once you get stronger.

lower back program

My general rule of thumb with back rehab is to start with stabilization exercises. That is, exercises where the main goal is to *not* move the spine. This way, you are isometrically strengthening all the spine stabilizers (the abdominals as well as all the deep muscles in between the vertebrae), but are not doing any damage whatsoever to the injured area because you are not moving it. Most of the exercises listed in the Lower Back Program are stabilization exercises or gentle spinal articulation exercises; they should be safe if you have a back injury. Experiment with Phase 1 exercises and select those that benefit you.

For Phase 2 of this program, start with all the Essential exercises; this should take you about 20 minutes and you should do the program at least 3 times a week to feel the benefits. Once you gain strength, add in the rest of the Supplemental exercises so that you are doing between 20–45 minutes each time you lay down.

Once you are out of pain, you can slowly add in some of the other exercises in the Target Workouts section, and see if you can stay out of pain. Eventually, the goal is to be able to do any of the workouts that you fancy, pain-free.

Sciatic Pain

If you have pain shooting down the side or back of your leg, make sure to do the glutes/rotator release on the roller or pinkie ball as well as the 3-way hip stretch. This kind of pain is due to an impinged sciatic nerve, which runs through the piriformis muscle (a hip rotator). Sometimes releasing and stretching the rotators and stretching along the nerve pathway can help alleviate this pain.

Sacral Pain

The sacrum is located at the base of the spine, where the glutes and rotators are attached. If you suffer from nagging pain in this area, try the Glutes and Rotators Release on the roller or pinkie ball and see if this helps.

LOWER BACK PHASE 1: Release/Stretch

PAGE		PROP	EXERCISE
70, 138		roller, pinkie ball	IT band release
72, 137		roller, pinkie ball	glutes and rotators release
100, 133		band, circle	3-way hip stretch

LOWER BACK PHASE 2: Strengthen

PAGE		PROP	EXERCISE
101		circle	deep abdominal cue
102		circle	upper abdominal curls
122		circle	bridge
112		circle	single-leg stretch
49–50		roller	supine stabilization series
76–77		band	supine leg series
75		band	single-leg circles
51		roller	bridge (and single-leg bridge)*
54		roller	knee stretch flat back*
52		roller	plank*

*Supplemental exercises

shoulder program

The following workout can address both acute injuries, such as a traumatic bike accident that dislocates your shoulder, and chronic conditions that arise from one too many power yoga classes that caused microtears in your rotator cuff. Tight chest muscles and a weak back can also contribute to chronic conditions such as rounded or rolled-forward shoulders, which cause misalignment of the shoulder joint. Phase 1 addresses tightness while Phase 2 deals with weakness.

Acute injuries: If you suffer from instability of the shoulder or have an acute injury, skip Phase 1 and go straight to Phase 2. For the Rotator Strengthener in the Shoulder Series, try this one arm at a time, and do an extra set or two on the weaker side.

Chronic conditions: You are free to do both phases.

If you're not sure of your condition, you can try the Basic Shoulder Set on the floor instead of the roller for a less intense version, and do the Pec Release instead of the 3-way Pec Stretch.

The Phase 2 exercises should take about 20 minutes to complete. If you are unstable, do 3 sets of 10, resting in between, at least once a day, every day. Once you get stronger, you can reduce your frequency to 3 times a week.

THE SHOULDERS PHASE 1: Release/Stretch

PAGE		PROP	EXERCISE
44–48		roller	basic shoulder set
91		band	3-way pec stretch
139		pinkie ball	pec release

THE SHOULDERS PHASE 2: Strengthen

PAGE		PROP	EXERCISE
91–94		band	shoulder series
85–88		band	lunging series*
129		circle	lat press*

Supplemental exercises

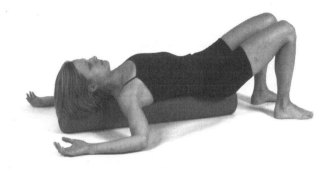

knee program

Phase 1 of this program is basically reserved for those people who have lateral knee pain, especially after bicycling or running. Try the IT Band Release before doing your strengthening exercises. Otherwise, if you don't suffer from lateral knee pain, skip this phase and go straight to Phase 2.

There are two specific muscles that are crucial in stabilizing the knee. The *Vastus Medialis Obliquus* (or VMO) is part of the quadriceps and very important to strengthen after a knee injury. Because it is responsible for the last few degrees of knee extension, it becomes atrophied almost immediately after injury because inflammation stops the knee from extending. Once the VMO has atrophied, the knee will become more unstable, which creates a negative spiral of potentially further injury to the knee. Also, the VMO is responsible for pulling the patella (knee cap) toward the inner thigh during the final phase of knee extension; strengthening it can correct improper tracking of the patella.

The *hamstrings* are the most important muscles to strengthen if you have an Anterior Cruciate Ligament (ACL) injury. The ACL is responsible for keeping the tibia stable on the femur; when the ACL is damaged, the tibia can move forward on the femur (like a drawer)—definitely not good for the knee.

THE KNEES PHASE 1: Release/Stretch

PAGE		PROP	EXERCISE
70, 138		roller, pinkie ball	IT band release

THE KNEES PHASE 2: Strengthen

PAGE		PROP	EXERCISE
96		band	quads (VMO) strengthener
97		band	hamstrings strengthener
99		band	abductor strengthener
98		band	adductor strengthener
76–77		band	supine leg series*
49		roller	tiny steps*
51		roller	bridge (and single-leg bridge)*
126–27		circle	side lying series*
130–32		circle	standing series*

*Supplemental exercises

Start with the Essential exercises (once you're stronger, add the Supplemental ones). For each exercise, do 3 sets of 10, resting in between sets, 3 times a day, every day. Each session will take 15–20 minutes. As you gain strength, you can reduce your workouts to 3 days a week until you no longer need to do them.

foot & ankle program

Foot Problems

The exercises here relieve foot or arch pain by strengthening the intrinsic muscles of your feet. They also can help bring the arch back in flat feet. Heel pain is the gold standard for plantar fasciitis, inflammation of the connective tissue of the foot. Releasing that tissue with Phase 1, as well as stretching your calf, can help stop the pain.

Do all the exercises in this program once a day to begin, and as your feet gain strength and you feel less pain, do the exercises 3 times a week before eventually tapering off.

Ankle Weakness

Once you've sprained your ankle, you have overstretched the ligaments and tendons, and are more susceptible to reinjury and chronic ankle instability. This program will help you strengthen and rebalance the muscles that need to compensate for lack of integrity. Lack of stability at the pelvic level also contributes to frequent ankle injury; the standing exercises help promote lower-limb stability from hips to ankle. Do Phase 1 and the Essential Phase 2 exercises once a day. You should also walk on your toes then heels for 1 minute a day. Add the Supplemental exercises once you get stronger. As you gain stability, drop down to 3 days a week, then eventually taper off.

THE FOOT PHASE 1: Release/Stretch

PAGE		PROP	EXERCISE
136		pinkie ball	foot release
58		roller	log roll

THE FOOT PHASE 2: Strengthen

135		small ball	short foot
95		band	foot and ankle strengthener
141		towel	the towel

THE ANKLE PHASE 1: Release/Stretch

PAGE		PROP	EXERCISE
136		pinkie ball	foot release

THE ANKLE PHASE 2: Strengthen

95		band	foot and ankle strengthener
59		roller	around the world
58		roller	log roll
130		circle	first/fourth position plies
98		band	adductor strengthener
99		band	abductor strengthener
135		small ball	short foot*
51		roller	bridge (and single-leg bridge)*
132		circle	single-leg standing lowers*

Supplemental exercises

neck & upper back program

Everyone who has worked at a computer for more than four hours at a time has probably experienced nagging neck and upper back tension. The reason for this is that the upper trapezius muscles, which run from the base of your skull to the tops of the shoulders, and other back and neck muscles become overly taxed when the arms are suspended for long periods of time.

The exercises in Phase 1 will work out existing knots and allow the affected muscles to relax. The Basic Shoulder Set on the roller is by far the most essential of all the exercises in this program. If you do nothing else, do this.

If you have more time, add in the strengthening exercises of Phase 2 to help keep your posture strong, your chest open, and your shoulders open and properly aligned. Do this program once a day.

Keep in mind that if you work at a computer or do activities that contribute to ongoing neck and upper back pain, you may have to continue with this program indefinitely.

NECK/UPPER BACK PHASE 1: Release/Stretch

PAGE		PROP	EXERCISE
44–48		roller	basic shoulder set
69		roller	upper back release
139		pinkie ball	trap release
140		pinkie ball	back "spot knot" release
91		band	3-way pec stretch

NECK/UPPER BACK PHASE 1: Strengthen

PAGE		PROP	EXERCISE
92		band	rhomboids strengthener
94		band	chest expansion
92		band	rotator strengthener
88		band	lunging rhomboids*
134		circle	chin squeeze*

*Supplemental exercises

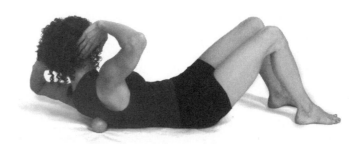

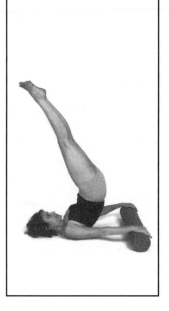

daily workouts

If you're wondering how you can utilize Pilates and props in your fitness plan, check out these full-body and targeted workouts. Choose a workout that suits your personal goals, depending on your time frame, level, and vanity needs.

How long do I have to work out to see results?

Twenty minutes is the minimum I would allocate to any workout regime. If you really want to see changes in your body, try 30–45 minutes each time. It's always better to do a shorter workout than not to do any at all, which is why I have engineered short bite-size workouts that you can combine to focus on the areas that you really want to strengthen.

How many times a week?

Twice a week is the absolute minimum to see changes in your body; 3–5 is the ideal. If you are a Type A personality, you will do no harm by doing a workout 7 days a week.

Balanced Full-Body Workouts on Each Prop

The following are three classic, Pilates-style workouts for these props: magic circle (or small

FULL-BODY WORKOUT TIME FRAME			
	CIRCLE	**BAND**	**ROLLER**
BEGINNING	30 min.	20 min.	25 min.
INTERMEDIATE	40 min.	30 min.	35 min.
ADVANCED	45 min.	35 min.	40 min.

ball), exercise band, and roller. To give your entire body a great workout, simply choose your prop and skill level:

- **BEGINNING:** Simply do all the beginning-level exercises in the listed order.
- **INTERMEDIATE:** Do all the beginning and intermediate exercises in the given order.
- **ADVANCED:** Do every exercise in the order listed for a killer workout. Though only the Magic Circle Workout offers a variety of specific, advanced-level moves, many of the exercises in the other workouts have advanced-level variations; you may choose to do these

instead of the beginning or intermediate versions.

Targeted Workouts

For those of you with limited time or more specific goals in mind, I've broken down the full-body workouts into a variety of subcategories:

- arms & legs
- articulation (to gain movement in your spine)
- butt & thighs
- core & arms
- core & legs
- core moves
- lengthening (to lengthen the spine)
- relax & release

- standing (to integrate the Pilates workout)
- standing balance
- stretch & extend

Refer to the workout chart for your selected prop and do all the prescribed exercises for your chosen target area at your skill level. For instance, beginners seeking to tone the buttocks and thighs using the magic circle should do all the "Butt & Thighs" routines listed (the Charlie Chaplin, Side Lying Series, and Bridge). If time and prop availability permit, you may also include the "Butt &

Thighs" routine from the Roller Workout (Squats against the Wall). Or you can pair "Core Moves" with "Stretch & Extend" for a completely different workout. The combinations are limitless—have fun!

Multiprop Workout

Using a prop in your Pilates workout is great, but using more than one is even better, allowing you to stimulate and tone your body in a multitude of ways.

Each prop has qualities that enhance the effect of Pilates mat-

work in their own special way, and for the Multiprop Workout, I've chosen the best exercises for each prop.

- **BEGINNING:** Simply do all the beginning-level exercises in the listed order. *Allow 20 minutes.*
- **INTERMEDIATE:** Do all the beginning and intermediate exercises in the given order. *Allow 30 minutes.*
- **ADVANCED:** Do every exercise in the order listed for a killer workout, using the advanced-level variation when available. *Allow 40 minutes.*

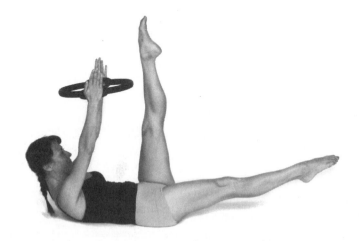

MAGIC CIRCLE WORKOUT

PAGE		EXERCISE	ROUTINE	LEVEL
122		bridge	warm-up	beginning
102		upper abdominal curls	warm-up	beginning
104		the hundred	warm-up	intermediate
106		roll-up	core moves	intermediate
103		single-leg roll-up	core moves	intermediate
107		rollover	core moves	advanced
110		rolling like a ball	core moves	beginning
120		hinge curl roll-down	core moves	advanced
123		around the world	core moves	intermediate
112–17		classic abs series	core moves	beginning–intermediate
124		double-leg kicks	butt & thighs	intermediate
125		charlie chaplin	butt & thighs	beginning
126–27		side lying series	butt & thighs	beginning
118		spine stretch forward	stretch & extend	beginning
111		straight-leg rocker	stretch & extend	advanced
119		swan	stretch & extend	beginning
133		3-way hip stretch	stretch & extend	beginning
128		pec squeeze	standing	beginning
130		first/fourth position plies	standing	intermediate

EXERCISE BAND WORKOUT

PAGE		EXERCISE	ROUTINE	LEVEL
76–77		supine leg series	warm-up	beginning
78		long spine stretch	warm-up	advanced
75		single-leg circles	core moves	beginning
73–74		roll-down with variations	core moves	beginning–intermediate
80–81		teaser series	core moves	beginning–advanced
84		doggie kick	butt & spine	beginning
84		FTD florist	butt & spine	intermediate
85–88		lunging series	arms & legs	beginning–intermediate
89–90		standing series	lengthening	beginning–intermediate
91		3-way pec stretch	cool down	beginning
100		3-way hip stretch	cool down	beginning

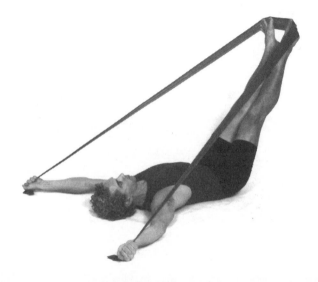

ROLLER WORKOUT

PAGE		EXERCISE	ROUTINE	LEVEL
44–48		basic shoulder set	relax & release	beginning
49–50		supine stabilization series	warm-up	beginning
67		swan	stretch & extend	beginning
51		bridge	extension	beginning
52–55		plank series	core & arms	intermediate–advanced
56		jackknife supine	core moves	advanced
60–65		supine leg series	core moves	beginning
66		squats against the wall	butt & thighs	beginning
58		log roll	standing balance	intermediate
59		around the world	standing balance	intermediate

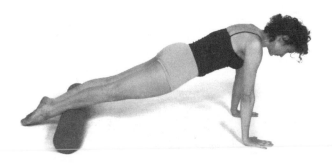

MULTIPROP WORKOUT

PAGE		EXERCISE	ROUTINE	LEVEL
44–48		basic shoulder set	relax & release	beginning
49–50		supine stabilization series	warm-up	beginning
122		bridge	warm-up	beginning
102		upper abdominal curls	warm-up	beginning
104		the hundred	warm-up	intermediate
103		single-leg roll-up	articulation	intermediate
133		3-way hip stretch	articulation	beginning
109		teaser into open-leg rocker	articulation	advanced
111		straight-leg rocker	articulation	advanced
52–55		plank series	core & arms	intermediate–advanced
112		single-leg stretch	core moves	beginning
113		double-leg stretch	core moves	intermediate
114		double-leg lowers	core moves	intermediate
116		criss cross	core moves	intermediate
117		scissors	core moves	intermediate
124		double-leg kicks	butt & thighs	intermediate
125		charlie chaplin	butt & thighs	beginning
126–27		side lying series	butt & thighs	beginning
76–77		supine leg series	core & legs	beginning
73		roll-down	articulation	beginning
85–88		lunging series	arms & legs	beginning–intermediate
89–90		standing series	lengthening	beginning–intermediate

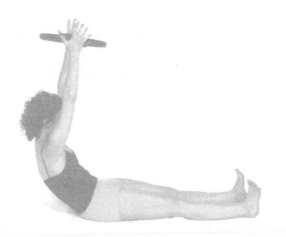

part three:
the
exercises

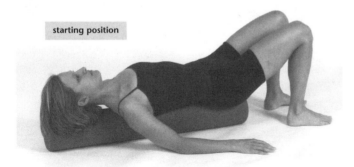

starting position

STARTING POSITION: Lie on your back so that the roller is under your spine, supporting you from head to tail. Place your feet a little wider than hip distance apart. Your arms should be down by your sides, palms facing down.

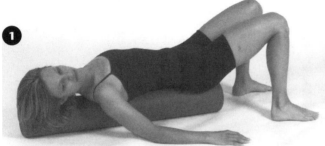

1

1—2 **INHALE AND EXHALE CONTINUOUSLY**: Rock from side to side, trying to initiate the movement from your center, keeping your navel pulled in toward your spine. Let your head look in the opposite direction of your body. Let the rocking become easy, rhythmic, and relaxed.

repeat for 1 minute

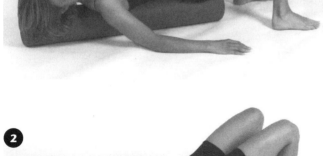

2

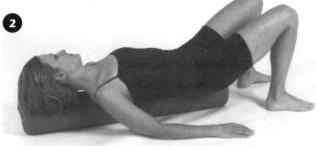

BENEFITS	DOS & DON'TS	IMAGINE
■ Opens the chest and pecs. ■ Releases neck and upper back tension. ■ Realigns the shoulders, neck, and head.	■ Do allow the neck to relax. ■ Do use your hands and feet to help you stabilize. ■ Don't roll so far to either side that you feel off-balance—no need to go to your "endpoint."	■ You are lying on a boat in the Caribbean, being lulled into a state of total relaxation.

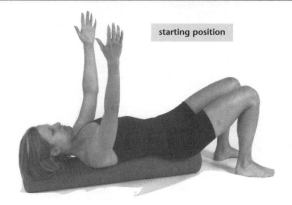

starting position

STARTING POSITION: Lie on your back so that the roller is under your spine, supporting you from head to tail. Place your feet a little wider than hip distance apart. Reach your arms up to the sky, palms facing each other.

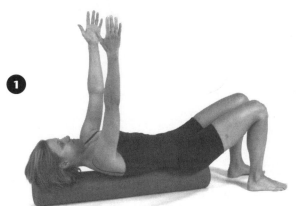

1 **INHALE**: Reach your arms up to the sky, allowing your shoulder blades (scapulas) to come off the roller.

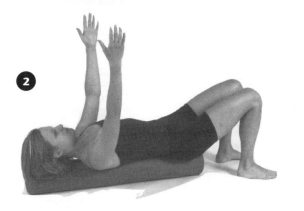

2 **EXHALE**: Keep the arms straight as you completely re-lax and release the shoulder mus-cles, letting the scapulas "slap" back down. On the final repetition, allow the scapulas to come down slowly, imagining the shoulder blades melting back into the roller and melting down away from your ears.

repeat | **4 times**

BENEFITS	DOS & DON'TS	IMAGINE
■ Releases tension in the shoulders, upper back, and neck. ■ Realigns the shoulder girdle.	■ Do really release on the exhale, allowing the shoulder blades and arms to truly drop with gravity. ■ Don't bend your arms when you slap the blades down. Keep them long and strong.	■ You are letting all the tension release on every slap.

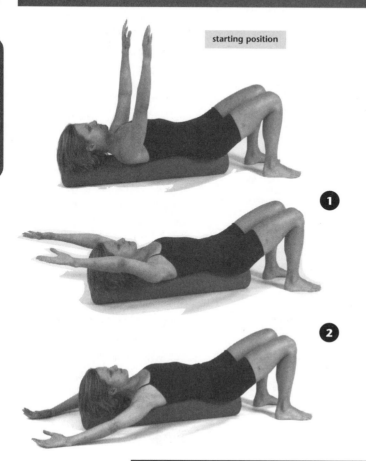

starting position

STARTING POSITION: Lie on your back so that the roller is under your spine, supporting you from head to tail. Place your feet a little wider than hip distance apart. Reach your arms up to the sky, palms facing forward. **INHALE TO BEGIN**.

1 EXHALE: On the first half of your exhale, think of knitting the ribs down, and then reach your arms back toward your ears. Feel the contact of your whole back on the roller; use the upper abdominals to keep the ribs down and to keep the upper back from arching off the roller.

2 INHALE: After four reps, drop the arms to the Deep Lat Stretch position.

repeat **4 times**

VARIATION

Arm Reaches with Magic Circle

Lie on your back with knees bent and feet flat on the floor, hip distance apart. Hold the magic circle between your hands and reach them up to the sky. Reach your arms back toward your ears, but only reach back as far as you can maintain the stabilization of your ribs.

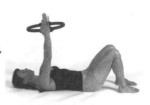

BENEFITS

- Stretches the lats and pecs.
- Teaches torso stabilization.
- Realigns the shoulder girdle.

DOS & DON'TS

- Do maintain absolute stability in the torso by keeping the ribs down.
- Do keep your shoulders down away from your ears as you initiate the exercise.
- Don't let your upper back arch off the roller. This is the whole point of this exercise because as you raise the arms, the upper back naturally wants to go with them.

IMAGINE

- Your arms originate from your back.

roller

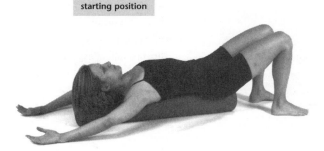

starting position

STARTING POSITION: Lie on your back so that the roller is under your spine, supporting you from head to tail. Place your feet a little wider than hip distance apart. Your arms are by your ears, reaching for the floor behind you, palms facing up. **INHALE TO BEGIN**.

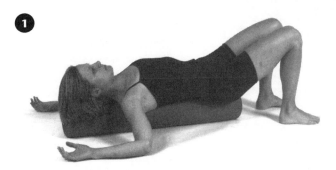

1 **EXHALE**: Start to slowly bend your elbows, pulling your elbows down as if aiming them for your back pockets. Try to keep the elbows bent at about a 90-degree angle as you do the exercise and try to let your elbows touch the floor. If you are very tight, they will not touch the floor, so just let them drop back as far as it feels comfortable. Imagine pulling your shoulder blades down your back with your back muscles.

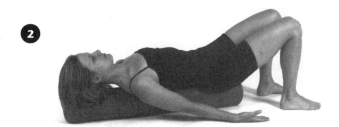

2 Once you've pulled your elbows down as far as you can, let your arms slowly straighten and come down by your sides.

Go right into Angels in the Snow (see next page).

repeat | 3–4 times with Angels in the Snow

BENEFITS	DOS & DON'TS	IMAGINE
▪ Stretches the pecs and chest muscles. ▪ Realigns the shoulder girdle. ▪ Engages the back muscles.	▪ Do breathe into the stretch. ▪ Do allow your chest to rise up off the roller if you are very tight.	▪ Your chest opens and expands each time you inhale.

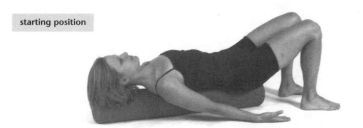

starting position

STARTING POSITION: Lie on your back so that the roller is under your spine, supporting you from head to tail. Place your feet a little wider than hip distance apart. Your arms are down by your sides, palms facing up. **INHALE TO BEGIN**.

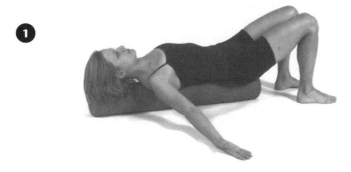

1–2 **EXHALE** and pull your shoulder blades down your back as you begin to drag your arms slowly along the floor. Continue breathing deeply as you open your arms to a "T" shape with your body. Keep the arms heavy on the floor to get a wonderful stretch in your chest as you continue moving the arms, completing the full arc of the angel wing when your arms end up by your ears.

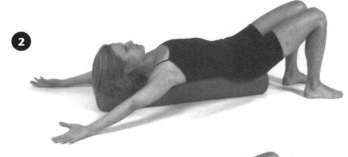

3 Do a Chicken Wing (see page 47) back down to return to starting position.

repeat **3 times**

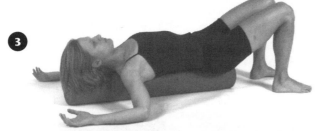

BENEFITS	DOS & DON'TS	IMAGINE
■ Stretches the pecs and chest muscles. ■ Realigns the shoulder girdle. ■ Teaches proper shoulder abduction.	■ Do hold the stretch at any place where you feel you need it. Breathe deeply to release. ■ Do keep your shoulders down away from your ears.	■ You are lying in the snow, pushing up the snow with your arms using your back muscles, allowing your chest to open and release.

roller

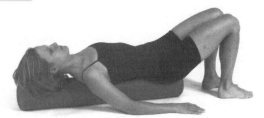

starting position

STARTING POSITION: Lie on your back so that the roller is under your spine, supporting you from head to tail. Bend your knees and place your feet flat on the floor about hip distance apart. Your arms are down by your sides, palms facing down. Feel free to press your arms into the floor to help you stabilize during this exercise. **INHALE TO BEGIN.**

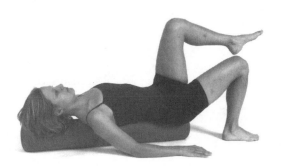

1 EXHALE: Pull the navel in toward the spine, flatten your low back onto the roller, and lift your left knee up to your chest. **INHALE:** Hold.

EXHALE: Still pulling in your navel to your spine, bring the left leg back down to the mat to the starting position, controlling the movement from the center.

repeat | 10 times alternating

VARIATIONS

Toe Taps   *intermediate*

Toe Taps is slightly more advanced than Tiny Steps because you never keep one foot planted for support; instead, keep your toes pointed and alternate tapping the mat with one foot as the other knee comes up to the chest. Breathe continuously as you tap, tap, tap, tap.

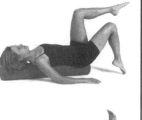

Taps with Flexed Feet
intermediate

Same as Toe Taps, but to increase the challenge, flex your feet and tap them to the mat.

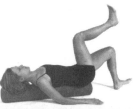

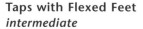

DOS & DON'TS

- Don't let your low back arch or your hips rock from side to side.

- Don't tense your upper body when doing this exercise. Keep your neck long and your shoulders relaxed.

IMAGINE

- You are lifting your leg from your lower spine.

starting position

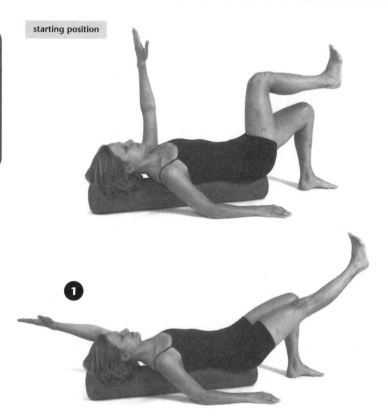

STARTING POSITION: Lie on your back so that the roller is under your spine, supporting you from head to tail. Bend your knees so that the left foot is flat on the floor and the right leg is up, knee bent at a right angle. Reach your left arm to the sky and your right arm down by your side, palm facing down. **INHALE TO BEGIN.**

1 EXHALE: Pull the navel in toward the spine. Flatten your low back onto the roller as you reach the left arm and right leg away from each other, keeping them in their own "tracks." Press through the heel of the right foot to straighten the leg away from the center.

INHALE: Bring the limbs back toward the center, returning to starting position.

| repeat | 8 times each side |

BENEFITS	DOS & DON'TS	IMAGINE
▪ Strengthens the core. ▪ Teaches torso stability.	▪ Do keep the whole spine in contact with the roller. ▪ Don't let the back arch off the roller or let the roller rock from side to side.	▪ You are pressing something away from you with your heel as you extend your leg.

starting position

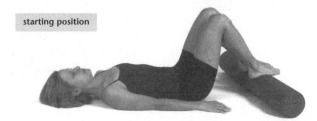

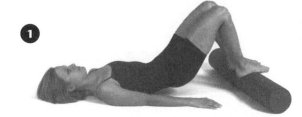

1

2

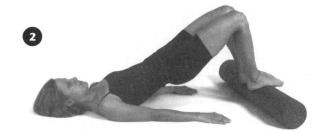

STARTING POSITION: Lie on your back with knees bent, hip distance apart, and feet standing on the roller. Your arms are down by your sides, palms facing down. **INHALE TO BEGIN**.

1 **EXHALE:** Pull the navel in toward the spine as you slowly roll your coccyx up off the mat, articulating through your spine until you are up in a Bridge.

2 Make sure your hips are lifted high enough that your body makes a straight diagonal line from shoulders to knees. **INHALE:** Hold Bridge for one full breath. **EXHALE** and pull the navel in toward the spine, squeezing your glutes, thinking of stretching through the front of your hips.

INHALE again, then **EXHALE** and return to starting position, rolling down one vertebra at a time.

repeat **6 times**

VARIATION

Single-leg Bridge   *intermediate*

Once up in the Bridge, exhale and take one leg off, lifting the knee toward the chest. Hold as you inhale, then on the exhale replace the leg on the roller. Lower your Bridge if it is too difficult to stabilize. Repeat 10 times, alternating sides. Keep your hips stable!

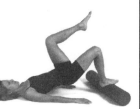

BENEFITS	DOS & DON'TS	IMAGINE
■ Strengthens the hamstrings and glutes. ■ Teaches spinal articulation.	■ Don't let the roller move. ■ Don't lift your hips so high that you arch your back. ■ Do press your door frame arms on the floor to help you stabilize.	■ You're keeping the log from rolling away with your core and hamstrings.

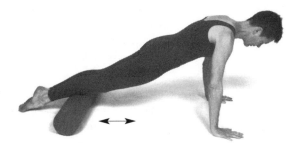

starting position

STARTING POSITION: Start with your shins on the roller. Your arms are shoulder distance apart, straight and strong, fingers spread, pressing away from the floor with your back muscles.

INHALE AND EXHALE CONTINU-OUSLY: Roll forward a few inches then roll back a few inches.

repeat **10 times**

VARIATION

beginning

Interlace your fingers. Place your forearms on the floor and open your elbows about shoulder distance apart. Press down through your forearms and try to create a little dome in your back, engaging your serratus anterior. This variation really helps strengthen and stabilize your shoulders, and is also a great alternative for those with wrist problems. Note also that the closer the roller is to your center, the less challenging the Plank will be.

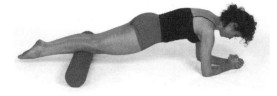

BENEFITS

- Strengthens the arms, back, and abdominals.
- Teaches balance.

DOS & DON'TS

- Do keep your body stable by engaging your powerhouse: pull the belly in, squeeze your butt, and pull your inner thighs together.

push-up

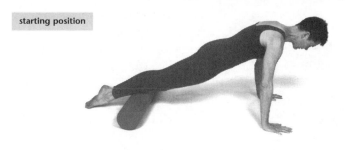

starting position

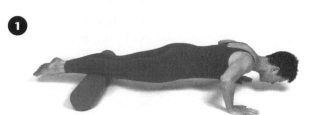

1

STARTING POSITION: Start in a Plank Position with your shins on the roller. Your arms are shoulder distance apart, straight and strong, fingers spread, pressing away from the floor with your back muscles. **INHALE TO BEGIN**.

1 **EXHALE:** Lower yourself to the ground, allowing your elbows to bend out to the sides.

INHALE and return to starting position.

repeat **10 times**

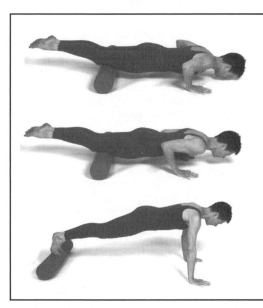

VARIATIONS

Push-up   *beginning*

Make the push-up easier by starting with the roller closer to your center, above the knees.

Triceps Push-up   *intermediate*

Keep your elbows in by your sides as you do this push-up. Make sure to keep your shoulders open; don't let them roll forward! Allow your chest to open to facilitate keeping the shoulders open.

Push-up   *advanced*

Start with your toes on the roller and feet flexed.

BENEFITS	DOS & DON'TS
■ Strengthens the arms, back, and abdominals. ■ Teaches balance.	■ Do keep your body stable by engaging your powerhouse: pull the belly in, squeeze your butt, and pull your inner thighs together.

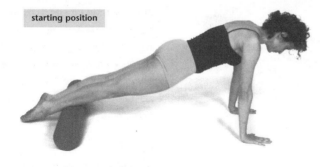

starting position

STARTING POSITION: Start in a Plank Position with the roller under your shins. Your arms are shoulder distance apart, straight and strong, fingers spread, pressing away from the floor with your back muscles. **INHALE TO BEGIN**.

1 EXHALE: Pull the roller in toward your arms, rounding your whole spine, creating a C-curve.

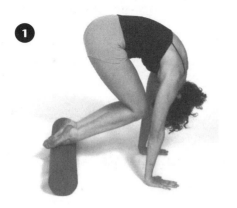

1

INHALE: Pull the navel in toward your spine as you extend your legs, sending the roller away from you, returning to starting position.

repeat	10 times

VARIATIONS

Knee Stretch Flat Back

Instead of creating a C-curve when you pull the roller in, keep your spine in Neutral, sending your tailbone backward (stick your butt out a little), still supporting the torso by pulling the navel in toward the spine.

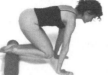

Knee Stretch on Elbows

If your wrists bother you, support yourself on your elbows with hands clasped. Push your forearms strongly into the mat to engage your back muscles as you pull the roller in.

BENEFITS	DOS & DON'TS	IMAGINE
■ Strengthens the arms, shoulders, back, and abdominals. ■ Stretches the spine.	■ Do keep your fingers spread and your arms straight and strong, pressing away from the floor using your back strength. ■ Don't extend your legs so far that you cannot maintain stability in your torso; if you feel any back strain, make the movement smaller.	■ You are pressing away from gravity.

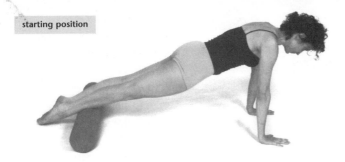

starting position

STARTING POSITION: Start in a Plank Position with your shins on the roller. Your arms are shoulder distance apart, straight and strong, fingers spread, pressing away from the floor with your back muscles. **INHALE TO BEGIN**.

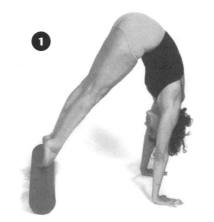

1

1 EXHALE: Fold your body in half by scooping your belly in toward your spine and pull the roller in toward your arms. Allow your head to follow the movement of the spine by dropping down so that you are looking at your knees.

INHALE and return to starting position.

repeat **8 times**

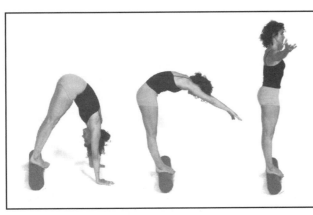

VARIATION

Jackknife Plank to Your Feet
super-advanced

This requires a great degree of core and upper body strength. At the top of your Jackknife, keep rolling the roller forward and lift up from your belly to get your feet to land on the roller with the arches planted. Then try to come up to standing by rolling up one vertebra at a time.

BENEFITS

- Strengthens the arms, back, and abdominals.
- Teaches inversion.

DOS & DON'TS

- Do keep your body stable by engaging your powerhouse: pull the belly in, squeeze your butt, and pull your inner thighs together.

- Do use the momentum to pull yourself as high as possible in your Jackknife.

roller

jackknife supine *advanced*

starting position

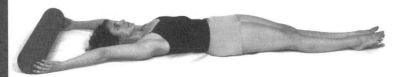

STARTING POSITION: Lie on your back and, holding the roller by the ends and keeping your upper back in contact with the floor, reach above your head, arms on the floor behind you. Your legs are also long on the floor in Pilates First Position. **INHALE TO BEGIN.**

1 Pull your navel in and keep your low back flat on the floor as you lift your arms and legs up to the sky.

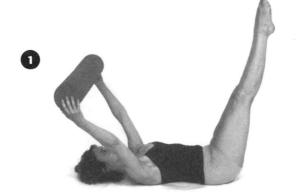

2 EXHALE: Scoop the belly in as you fold your body in half, lifting your hips up as you reach the roller forward and flexing your feet so you can slip them under the roller.

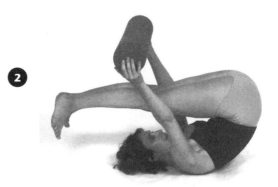

BENEFITS	DOS & DON'TS	IMAGINE
■ Strengthens the abdominals, butt, arms, and back. ■ Stretches the neck and upper back.	■ Make sure to maintain a flat low back when your legs drop away from your center on the first movement. Keep your belly absolutely scooped! ■ Don't roll up onto your neck—try to keep the weight balanced between your shoulder blades instead.	■ You are a spring-loaded jackknife.

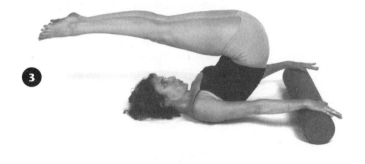

3 Place the roller on the floor beneath your hips, balancing between your shoulder blades.

4 Levitate your hips and legs upward, pressing down on the roller with your arms to give you extra lift and support. **INHALE** at the top. (Do not inhale at the top if you're worried about your neck.)

5–6 **EXHALE**: Retrograde the movement and return to starting position.

| repeat | 4 times |

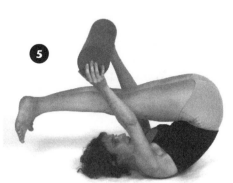

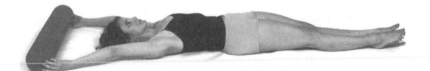

log roll

STARTING POSITION: Stand on the roller.

1–2 **INHALE AND EXHALE CONTINUOUSLY:**
Keeping the roller under your feet, walk in small steps across the room.

repeat	until you roll across the room

starting position

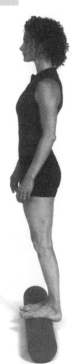

1

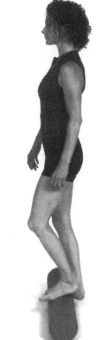

2

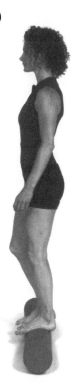

BENEFITS	DOS & DON'TS	IMAGINE
■ Teaches balance and stability. ■ Releases the fascia of the foot.	■ Don't do if you have a soft roller (it may smush the roller permanently). ■ Do keep the belly scooped in to help you balance.	■ You are a dancing bear in the circus.

STARTING POSITION: Stand on the roller with one foot and allow the other leg to hang in front of you, both knees soft. Stand next to a wall if you need support.

1 **INHALE AND EXHALE CONTINUOUSLY:** Hold the balance for 3 full breaths.

2–3 Start to move the free leg in all directions, extending it to the front, to the side, and finally to the back for an arabesque.

repeat	once each side

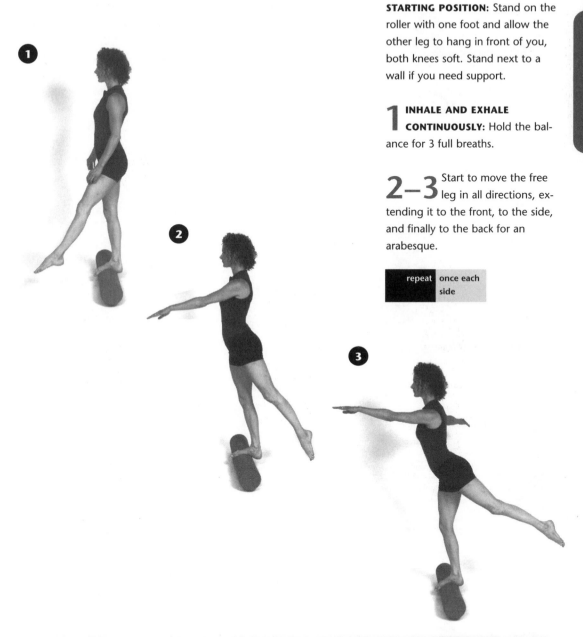

BENEFITS	DOS & DON'TS	IMAGINE
■ Teaches balance and stability. ■ Releases the fascia of the foot.	■ Don't do if you have a soft roller (it may smush the roller permanently). ■ Do keep the belly scooped in to help you balance.	■ Your balance originates from a line of energy starting from under the arch of the foot, rising up along the inner thigh line, and continues up into the abdominal core.

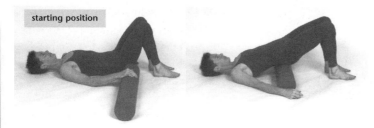

starting position

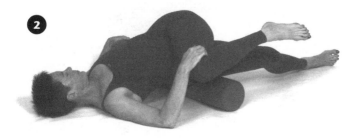

①

②

STARTING POSITION: Lie on your back with knees bent and feet flat on the floor. Lift your hips and slip the roller under your sacrum.

1 *Hip Flexor Stretch:* Bend one knee in toward your chest and extend the other leg out on the mat in front of you. Make sure your pelvis is tucked under by putting the roller as far down as possible on your tail. You can hold on to the side of the roller with one hand while you hold the knee with the other. **INHALE** and hold the stretch. **EXHALE** and pull your navel in toward your spine and squeeze your glute on the extended side to increase the hip flexor stretch. **INHALE**.

2 *Spine Twist:* **EXHALE**: Pull your navel to your spine and cross the bent knee over your body as far as you can. Some people go all the way to the floor. Breathe continuously for a few breaths and switch sides.

repeat once each side

BENEFITS	DOS & DON'TS	IMAGINE
■ *Hip Flexor Stretch:* Stretches the hip flexors. ■ *Spine Twist:* Stretches the spine, back muscles, and chest.	■ Don't strain your back. If you have a sensitive back, skip this exercise. ■ Don't let your low back arch; keep the navel pulling in toward your spine and tuck your pelvis under.	■ *Hip Flexor Stretch:* Your hip is stretching long in front. ■ *Spine Twist:* You are wringing out your spine like a wet towel.

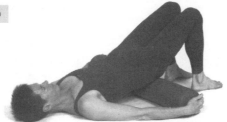

starting position

STARTING POSITION: Lie on your back with the roller under your sacrum, both knees bent, hip distance apart, feet flat on the floor. Make sure your pelvis is tucked under by putting the roller as far down as possible on your tail. Hold on to the sides of the roller with both hands to help you stabilize. **INHALE TO BEGIN**.

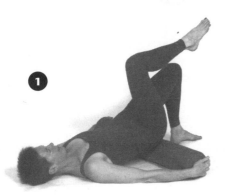

1

1 EXHALE: Pull your navel in toward your spine as you lift your right knee up to your chest.

INHALE: Bring the right foot back down to the mat to the starting position, controlling the movement from the center.

repeat	10 times alternating

VARIATIONS

Toe Taps   *beginning*

This is slightly more advanced than Tiny Steps because you never keep one foot planted for support; instead, keep your toes pointed and alternate tapping the mat with one foot as the other knee comes up to the chest. Breathe continuously as you tap, tap, tap, tap.

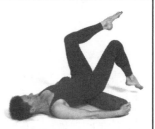

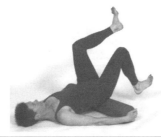

Taps with Flexed Feet   *beginning*

Same as Toe Taps above, but to increase the challenge, flex your feet and tap your heels to the mat.

BENEFITS	DOS & DON'TS	IMAGINE
▪ Strengthens the abdominals. ▪ Teaches torso stability.	▪ Don't let your low back arch or your hips rock from side to side. ▪ Don't tense your upper body when doing this exercise. Keep your neck long and your shoulders relaxed.	▪ Your thighs originate from your belly.

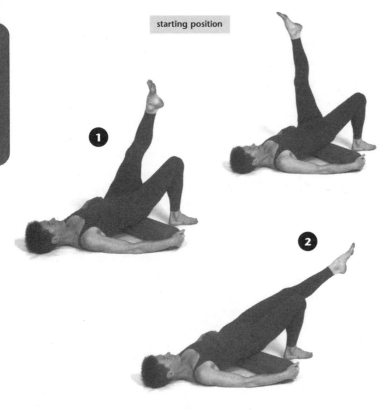

starting position

1

2

3

STARTING POSITION: Lie on your back with the roller under your sacrum, right knee bent with foot flat on the floor, left leg extended up to the sky. Make sure your pelvis is tucked under by putting the roller as far down as possible on your tail. Hold on to the sides of the roller with both hands to help you stabilize. **INHALE TO BEGIN.**

1–2 EXHALE AND INHALE:
Pull the navel in toward the spine and inscribe a long oval shape with your left big toe, first crossing the leg over the body then down toward the floor...

3 ...then a few inches outside of
the body and back up. Accent the "up" motion as you inhale.

repeat	3 times, switch directions; alternate sides

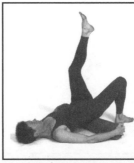

MODIFICATION
Try slightly bending the circling leg if you have tight hamstrings.

BENEFITS	DOS & DON'TS	IMAGINE
■ Strengthens the abdominals, especially the obliques. ■ Teaches hip freedom.	■ Do keep absolute stability in the torso by keeping your abdominal scoop. ■ Don't make the circle so big that you can't control the motion.	■ Your torso can stay absolutely stable while the leg moves freely.

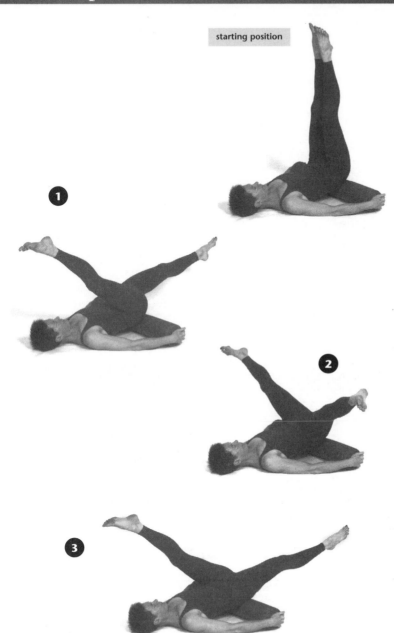

starting position

1

2

3

STARTING POSITION: Lie on your back with the roller under your sacrum. Extend both legs, reaching up toward the sky in Pilates First Position, externally rotated from the hip. Make sure your pelvis is tucked under by putting the roller as far down as possible on your tail. Hold on to the sides of the roller with your hands to help you stabilize.

1 INHALE AND EXHALE CONTINUOUSLY: Split the legs, reaching the right leg toward your head and the left leg down toward the floor.

2 Circle the left leg down and out to the side as the right leg comes up and out to the side.

3 As the left leg begins to circle back up, the right leg begins its circle in the opposite direction, opening it out to the right, then down toward the floor, then up through the center line. Reverse directions after every helicopter.

repeat 8 times

BENEFITS OF SUPINE LEG SERIES	DOS & DON'TS
■ Teaches coordination and torso stability. ■ Opens up the hips. ■ Strengthens the abdominals and inner thighs.	■ Do keep absolute stability in the torso by keeping your abdominal scoop. ■ Don't reach so far down with your legs that you can't keep your belly pulled in.

roller

bicycle *beginning*

starting position

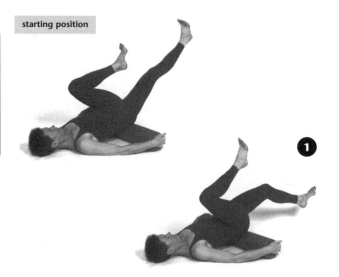

1

STARTING POSITION: Lie on your back with the roller under your sacrum, one knee bent up toward your chest, the other leg extended forward. Make sure your pelvis is tucked under. Hold on to the sides of the roller with both hands to help you stabilize.

1 **INHALE AND EXHALE CONTINUOUSLY:** Pedal the bent leg up and forward as the extended leg bends in toward the chest. Keep pedaling forward for 8 revolutions, then reverse directions and bicycle backward for 8 revolutions.

repeat	8 revolutions, forward and backward

scissors (changement) *beginning*

starting position

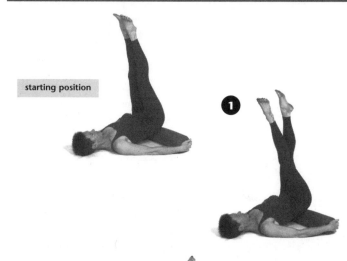

1

2

STARTING POSITION: Lie on your back with the roller under your sacrum. Extend both legs, reaching up toward the sky in Pilates First Position, externally rotated from the hip. Make sure your pelvis is tucked under. Hold on to the sides of the roller with both hands to help you stabilize. **INHALE TO BEGIN**.

1–2 **EXHALE:** Making small, quick beats, switch one foot in front of the other, reaching the legs incrementally down on 8 scissor beats.

INHALE: Come up for 8 scissor beats.

repeat	3 times

frog legs
beginning

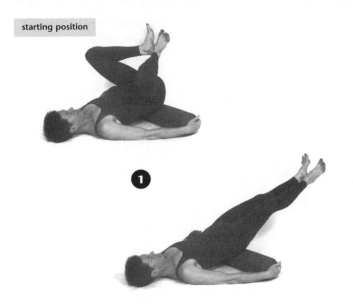

starting position

1

STARTING POSITION: Lie on your back with the roller under your sacrum. Your legs are off the floor in a frog squat, knees bent and turned out, feet flexed, heels pressing together. Make sure your pelvis is tucked under. Hold on to the sides of the roller with both hands to help you stabilize. **INHALE TO BEGIN.**

1 EXHALE: Pull the navel in toward your spine as you extend both legs diagonally, pulling your inner thighs together as you straighten your legs.

INHALE and return to frog squat.

repeat 8 times

double-leg circles
beginning

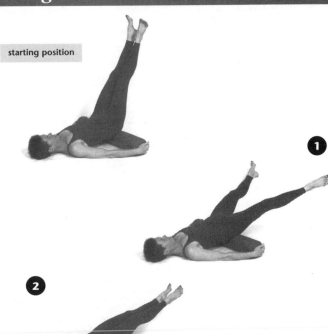

starting position

1

2

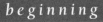

STARTING POSITION: Lie on your back with the roller under your sacrum. Extend both legs, reaching up toward the sky in Pilates First Position, externally rotated from the hip. Make sure your pelvis is tucked under. Hold on to the sides of the roller with both hands to help you stabilize. **INHALE TO BEGIN.**

1–2 EXHALE: Open the legs about twice as wide as your body and circle them down. Pull the inner thighs together at the bottom. **INHALE:** Keeping your legs firmly together, lift them up to starting position.

repeat 4 times, switch directions

roller

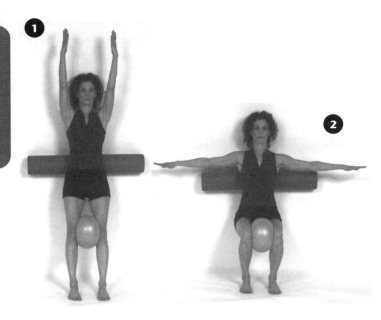

STARTING POSITION: Stand with your back to a wall, leaning against a horizontal roller underneath your low back. Your feet should be a couple of feet away from the wall with the small ball between your knees. You may adjust the distance once you try a squat. **INHALE TO BEGIN.**

1–2 EXHALE: Pull your navel in toward your spine and press into your heels as you bend your knees down into a squat. The roller will roll with you. Stick your butt out a little and lift your toes. Hold for one full breath.

INHALE and return to starting position.

repeat	5 times slowly then 10 times double time

VARIATION

Second Position

Repeat exercise with legs open and turned out from the hip. Keep the knee aligned over the middle toes.

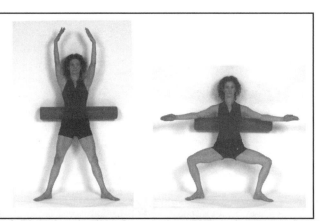

BENEFITS	**DOS & DON'TS**	**IMAGINE**
■ Strengthens the quads, butt, and hamstrings.	■ Do maintain neutral pelvis. ■ Don't bend your knees lower than 90 degrees. ■ Do maintain proper knee alignment, keeping the knee caps aligned over the second and third toes.	■ You are energetically lifting up as you go down.

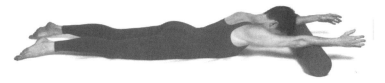

starting position

STARTING POSITION: Lie on your belly with your arms over your head, forearms resting on the roller, palms facing each other. Your head is slightly off the mat, eyes looking down. **INHALE TO BEGIN**.

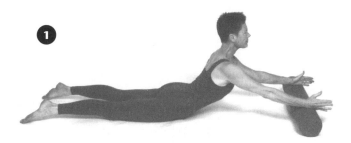

1

1 EXHALE: Pull the navel in toward the spine and gently engage your glutes by lengthening your pubic bone down onto the mat as you slowly pull the shoulder blades down the back, rolling the roller slightly toward you, rising up with your head, neck, and upper back into a spine extension, or Swan.

INHALE and retrograde the movement slowly, allowing the roller to roll away.

repeat 5 times

BENEFITS	DOS & DON'TS	IMAGINE
■ Strengthens the neck and back muscles. ■ Teaches proper shoulder, neck, and head alignment. ■ Reverses slumping posture.	■ Do really pull the belly in to protect the low back. ■ Don't come up so high that you strain your low back. ■ Don't break your Rosebud! Keep your head following the natural curve of your spine.	■ As you rise up to the Swan, you are watching an ant crawl away from you along the floor and eventually up the wall facing you. This will facilitate proper head alignment.

starting position

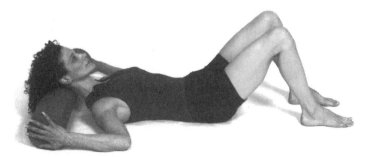

STARTING POSITION: Lie on your back with the roller under your neck, knees bent, feet flat on the floor. Hold on to the sides of the roller with both hands.

1 INHALE AND EXHALE CONTINUOUSLY: Roll your head slowly from side to side, feeling the delicious release in your neck.

repeat as needed

1

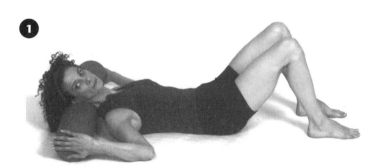

MODIFICATION

You can increase the stretch in your trapezius by bringing your chin down toward your chest once you've turned your head to one side.

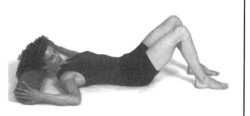

BENEFITS	DOS & DON'TS	IMAGINE
■ Releases the neck muscles.	■ Do adjust the position of the roller up and down the neck to get to your special tight places. ■ Do let the weight of your head release down into the roller.	■ You are saying "no" to neck pain.

roller

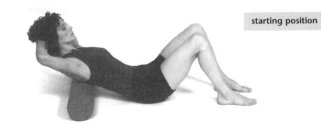

starting position

STARTING POSITION: Lie on your back, knees bent, feet flat on the floor, with the roller beneath your shoulder blades. Interlace your fingers behind your head. Start with your butt on the mat. **INHALE TO BEGIN**.

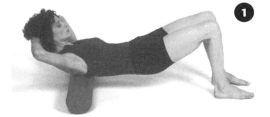

1 EXHALE: Press into your feet and lift your butt up.

2 INHALE: Gently arch your back, opening your chest and elbows, allowing the back muscles to get a massage.

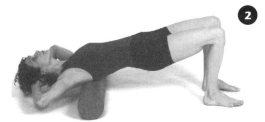

3 EXHALE: Gently round forward, bringing your head forward and creating a C-curve in your upper back.

repeat 5–10 times

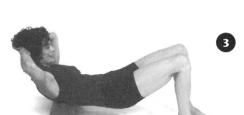

VARIATION

Self-Massage

Once your butt is up, try simply rolling back and forth along your upper back. Experiment with extending and flexing your spine to give yourself your own special massage.

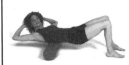

Try arcing to one side by bringing one elbow toward the hip on the same side; this opens up the opposite scapular area and allows for a deeper muscle release around the shoulder blades.

BENEFITS	DOS & DON'TS	IMAGINE
■ Releases the upper back muscles. ■ Teaches articulation and flexion in the thoracic spine.	■ Do keep your head supported by your hands; don't let it hang back. ■ Do support your hips by using your glutes to keep them lifted and by pulling your belly in.	■ You don't have to pay a masseuse every time you get a knot!

muscle releases
IT (iliotibial) band release
beginning

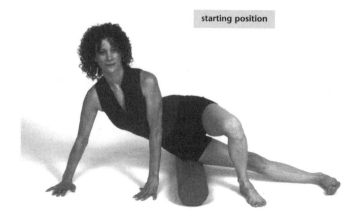

starting position

STARTING POSITION: Sit on the side of your hip with the roller underneath. The bottom leg is straight, with the side of the foot resting on the mat, and the top leg is bent with the foot in front. Your arms are straight and strong on the floor, supporting your body weight.

1 INHALE AND EXHALE CONTINUOUSLY: Roll up and down the side of your leg, making sure not to skip the area close to your knee. This is generally the tightest (thus the most painful) area of the IT band.

repeat | 30 seconds

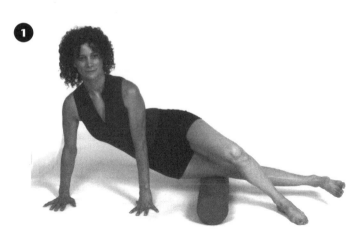

BENEFITS	DOS & DON'TS	IMAGINE
■ Releases the IT band (which can be the cause of lateral knee, hip, and back pain).	■ Don't stop just because its excruciating—often the tighter the IT band, the more it needs releasing. ■ Don't roll over the knee. ■ Do use your arm strength to modulate the amount of leg weight pressing into the roller.	■ The pain you are experiencing will put you in a good mood from all the endorphins!

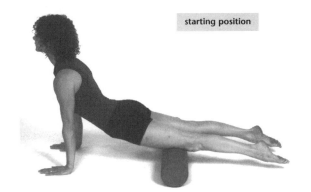

starting position

STARTING POSITION: Lie prone with your thighs on the roller. Your arms are supporting you in front, and you are lifted up in a High Swan. Don't hyperextend your low back as you come up into the Swan; instead, support the back by pulling the navel in toward your spine and gently squeezing your glutes.

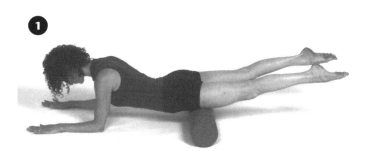

1

1 INHALE: Roll back toward the upper thighs as you bend the arms, bringing the elbows down to the mat. As you bend the elbows, keep proper shoulder alignment by keeping the elbows in by your sides and your shoulders rotating open.

EXHALE and return to starting position.

repeat **8 times**

VARIATION

Experiment with internally and externally rotating your legs to expose the inner and outer thighs to the roller.

BENEFITS	DOS & DON'TS	IMAGINE
▪ Releases the quads. ▪ Strengthens the arms, shoulders, glutes, and back. ▪ Teaches proper spine alignment.	▪ Do keep your head like a Rosebud on a stem, following the line of the spine—no broken buds! ▪ Don't roll over the knee. ▪ Do keep your shoulders down away from your ears as you straighten your arms.	▪ You are a toy Swan; your body keeps its Swan shape as you rock forward and back.

muscle releases

hamstrings release
intermediate

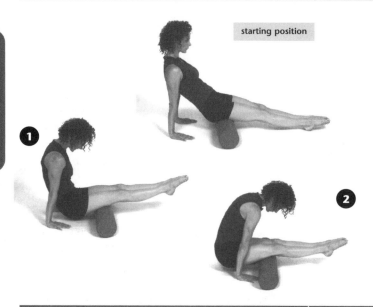

starting position

STARTING POSITION: Sit up with the backs of your thighs resting on the roller, arms supporting you from behind, fingers facing forward. **INHALE TO BEGIN.**

1–2 EXHALE: As the roller rolls down toward the knees, fold in half from the middle, lifting from your belly and pushing away from the floor with your arms.

INHALE and return to starting position.

repeat | 5–10 times

glutes and rotators release
beginning

STARTING POSITION: Sit on the roller on one hip, with that leg extended; the other knee is bent and open with the foot flat on the floor.

1–2 INHALE AND EXHALE CONTINUOUSLY: Start on the outside of your hip and roll slowly back and forth, allowing your weight to drop into the roller. Keep the back-and-forth roller motion as you slowly adjust your position, rolling slowly over the hip toward your spine, massaging all the different glutes and rotators along the way.

repeat | 30–60 seconds each side

BENEFITS	DOS & DON'TS	IMAGINE
■ *Hamstrings Release:* Releases the hamstrings; strengthens the arms, shoulders, and belly. ■ *Glutes and Rotators Release:* Releases the hip muscles.	■ Do enjoy the release, and focus on any area that feels tight.	■ *Hamstrings Release:* You are resisting gravity with your strong arms and back. ■ *Glutes and Rotators Release:* Your butt can actually relax.

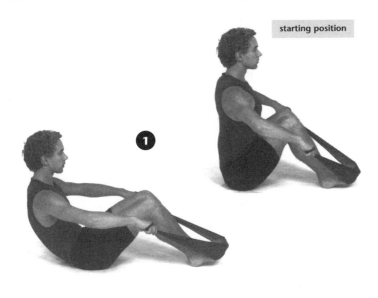

starting position

1

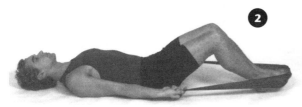

2

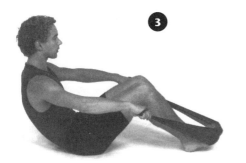

3

STARTING POSITION: Sit up on the mat with your knees bent in front of you. Wrap the exercise band around your feet and hold on to each end. Your elbows are slightly bent and open to the sides, your shoulders wide and relaxed down the back. **INHALE TO BEGIN** and lift your belly up off your hips, sitting tall.

1–2 EXHALE: Pull the navel in toward your spine and begin to roll down, creating a C-curve in your low back. Roll down one vertebra at a time until you are lying flat on your back. **INHALE** and hold. Turn your palms up and slide your scapulas down your back.

3 EXHALE: Squeeze a Tangerine under your chin to lift your head, then roll back up in your C-curve, making sure to scoop the belly in and press your low back onto the mat as you roll up. **INHALE:** Stack up from the base of your spine, the head being the last thing to rise.

EXHALE: Let your shoulders drop down the back and return to starting position.

repeat **5 times**

BENEFITS	DOS & DON'TS	IMAGINE
■ Strengthens the abdominals and the hip and neck flexors. ■ Teaches C-curve and articulation of the spine.	■ Do allow the exercise band to assist you by thinking of stretching your spine as you roll down. ■ Do keep your neck relaxed and your shoulders down your back.	■ You are imprinting your vertebrae onto a sandy beach beneath you.

VARIATIONS

Biceps Curl Roll-down   *intermediate*

Start the roll-down with knees bent, but stop about halfway down (when your low back is pressing on the mat) and breathe continuously as you bend the elbows against the resistance, keeping your elbows glued in to your sides. Repeat 8 Biceps Curls and then complete the roll-down exercise.

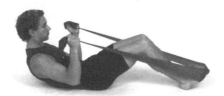

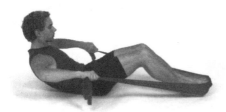

Rhomboid Pull Roll-down   *beginning*

Start the roll-down with knees bent, but stop about halfway down (when your low back is pressing on the mat) and breathe continuously as you bend the elbows against the resistance, keeping your elbows wide and pulling back behind you. Repeat 8 Rhomboid Pulls and then complete the roll-down exercise.

Oblique Roll-down   *beginning*

To emphasize the oblique abdominals, once you are down in your C-curve, with your low back imprinted on the mat, turn to one side with your upper torso. Open the arms, pulling away from the body, then come back to center and turn to the other side and open the arms. Repeat 8 times, alternating sides.

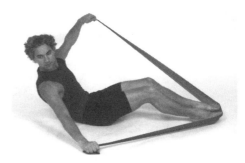

Pearl Button Roll-down   *intermediate*

Exhale to start the roll-down, but stop about halfway down, when your low back is pressing on the mat, and inhale. On the next exhale, roll down one vertebra and stop. Repeat this stop-and-start movement for 4 more breaths, using the exhale to articulate the spine, rolling down as if you are pressing the "pearl buttons" on your cardigan into the mat beneath you. Once you are flat on your back, inhale and hold. Try to retrograde the same sequence coming back up. Finish by stacking up the spine.

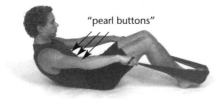

"pearl buttons"

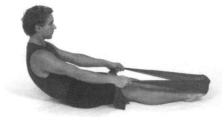

Straight-leg Roll-down   *intermediate*

To increase the difficulty of the roll-down, keep your legs extended in from of you. Repeat 5 times.

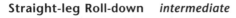

exercise band

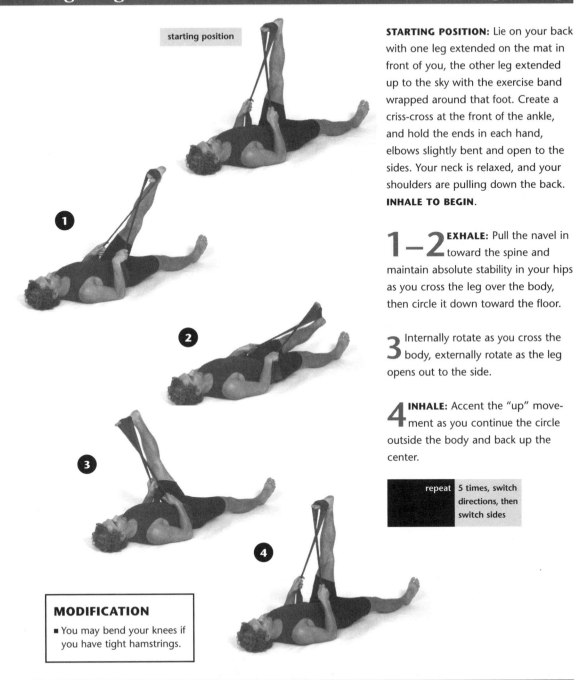

starting position

1

2

3

4

STARTING POSITION: Lie on your back with one leg extended on the mat in front of you, the other leg extended up to the sky with the exercise band wrapped around that foot. Create a criss-cross at the front of the ankle, and hold the ends in each hand, elbows slightly bent and open to the sides. Your neck is relaxed, and your shoulders are pulling down the back. **INHALE TO BEGIN**.

1−2 **EXHALE:** Pull the navel in toward the spine and maintain absolute stability in your hips as you cross the leg over the body, then circle it down toward the floor.

3 Internally rotate as you cross the body, externally rotate as the leg opens out to the side.

4 **INHALE:** Accent the "up" movement as you continue the circle outside the body and back up the center.

repeat	5 times, switch directions, then switch sides

exercise band

MODIFICATION
- You may bend your knees if you have tight hamstrings.

BENEFITS	DOS & DON'TS	IMAGINE
■ Strengthens the abdominals, especially the obliques. ■ Teaches pelvic stability.	■ Don't let your hips rock from side to side. ■ Do keep your neck relaxed.	■ Your pelvis is pinned to the mat by two stakes, each right inside your hip bones.

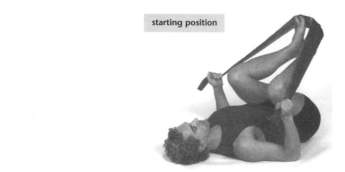

starting position

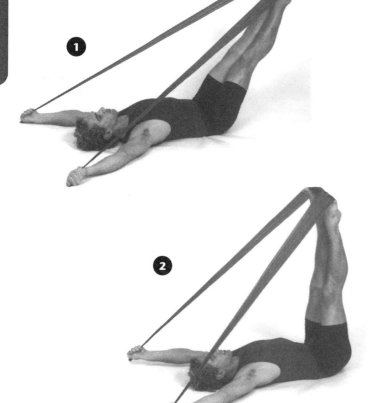

1

2

STARTING POSITION: Lie on your back with the exercise band wrapped around your feet. Hold the ends of the exercise band in your hands. **INHALE TO BEGIN**.

1 Extend your legs in Pilates First Position, toes slightly apart, heels together, inner thighs squeezing together as you extend the arms above your head on the floor behind you. **EXHALE**: Scoop your belly in, keeping a flat low back on the mat as you lower your legs toward the floor. Simultaneously extend your arms diagonally back by your ears.

2 **INHALE**: Keeping the arms extended by your ears, lift the legs back up so that they make a 90-degree angle with the floor.

repeat 8 times

MODIFICATIONS

- Always modify any exercise with the legs supported in front of you by keeping them lifted rather than close to the floor. This makes it easier for the abdominals to stabilize and maintain a flat low back.

BENEFITS	DOS & DON'TS	IMAGINE
■ Strengthens the core muscles.	■ Do keep your belly scooped. ■ Don't arch your back off the mat.	■ Your legs reach far and away.

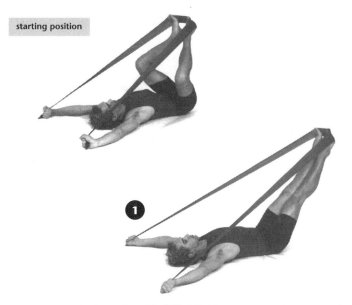

starting position

STARTING POSITION: Begin in a frog squat. Extend your arms diagonally back by your ears. **INHALE TO BEGIN**.

1 **EXHALE:** Scoop your belly in, keeping a flat low back on the mat as you extend the legs straight diagonally.

INHALE and return to starting position.

repeat 8 times

exercise band

dolphin | *beginning*

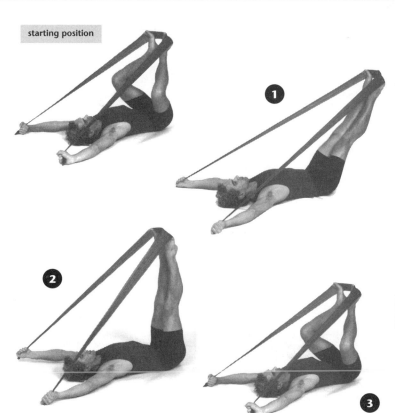

starting position

Dolphin is a combination of Leg Pulls and Frog Legs.

STARTING POSITION: Begin in a frog squat. Extend your arms diagonally back by your ears. **INHALE TO BEGIN**.

1 **EXHALE:** Extend your legs diagonally, keeping your low back flat on the mat.

2–3 **INHALE:** Lift your legs until they're 90 degrees to the floor, then pull them down into a frog squat.

repeat 8 times then reverse

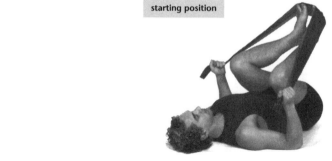

starting position

1

2

STARTING POSITION: Lie on your back with your legs in a frog squat. Wrap the exercise band around your feet and hold the ends in your hands, elbows bent and glued in to your sides. **INHALE TO BEGIN**.

1 Scoop your belly in, keeping your low back flat on the mat as you extend your legs diagonally and your arms up over your head on the mat behind you.

2 **EXHALE:** Scoop your belly in as you lift your legs up and over you, levitating your hips as if a hot spatula slid underneath your butt. Make a "J" shape with your whole body. Assist the movement by extending your arms back to the floor above your head, pulling your legs with the exercise band. **INHALE:** Balance between your shoulder blades; don't roll onto your neck.

BENEFITS	DOS & DON'TS	IMAGINE
■ Strengthens the abdominals, glutes, and hamstrings. ■ Stretches the spine.	■ Don't roll onto your neck. Instead, balance between your shoulder blades.	■ Your body is making a capital "J."

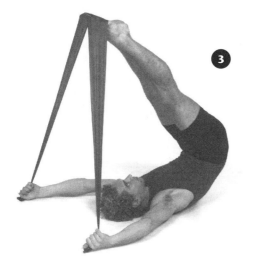

3 **EXHALE**: Maintain the "J" shape as you roll down your spine, keeping your hips as lifted as possible on the way down. As you repeat the exercise, keep the arms extended above the head.

4 Drop the legs back to the diagonal, keeping a flat low back and scooped-in belly.

INHALE and return to starting position.

repeat | 4 times

exercise band

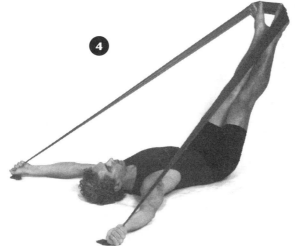

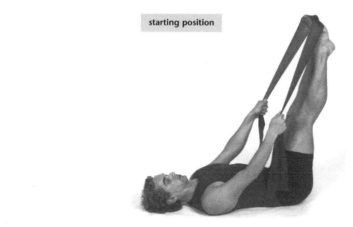

starting position

STARTING POSITION: Lie on your back with your legs extended to up to the sky, inner thighs squeezing together, feet turned out in Pilates First Position, toes slightly apart, heels together. Wrap the exercise band around your feet and hold the ends in your hands, arms extended forward, with some tension on the exercise band. **INHALE TO BEGIN.**

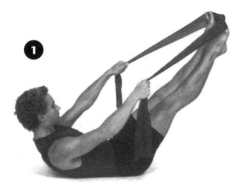

1–2 EXHALE: Allow your shoulder blades to pull down your back as you Squeeze a Tangerine under your chin to lift your head and roll up to the Teaser position. Balance just behind your tailbone, with your low belly scooped in and your low back slightly rounded. The exercise band can assist you in this by allowing your elbows to bend and open to the sides, increasing the tension on the exercise band as you roll up. **INHALE:** Lift the chest and hold.

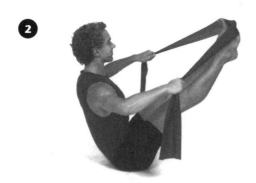

EXHALE: Roll down one vertebra at a time and return to the starting position.

repeat **6 times**

BENEFITS	DOS & DON'TS	IMAGINE
■ Strengthens the abdominals, hip flexors, and neck flexors.	■ Do keep the shoulders down away from the ears. ■ Do try to keep your legs stable as you roll up and down.	■ Why this exercise is called Teaser.

diamond-leg teaser *intermediate*

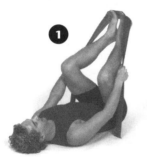 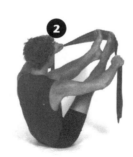

STARTING POSITION: Lie on your back with your legs in a frog squat. Wrap the exercise band around your feet and hold the ends in your hands, arms extended forward, with some tension on the band. **INHALE TO BEGIN**.

1 **EXHALE:** Squeeze a Tangerine under your chin to lift your head and roll up to the Teaser position. Do the Teaser, keeping the knees bent and open to a diamond shape, feet flexed and heels squeezing together.

repeat 5 times

dead-hang teaser *super-advanced*

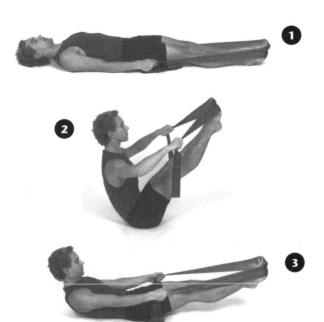

STARTING POSITION: Lie on your back with your legs straight on the floor. Wrap the band around your feet and hold the ends in your hands. **INHALE TO BEGIN**.

1–2 **EXHALE:** Squeeze a Tangerine under your chin to lift your head and roll up to the Teaser position.

3 When you come down, let the legs slowly drop to the dead hang position. Make sure you can keep your low back flat on the mat with your legs low.

repeat 5 times

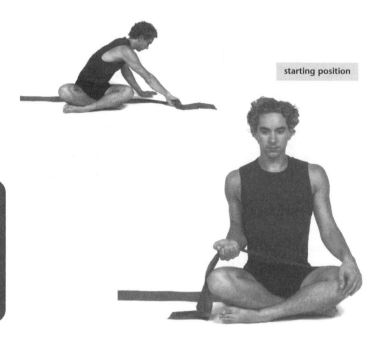

starting position

STARTING POSITION: Sit cross-legged on the middle of the exercise band. Pick up one end of the exercise band with the opposite hand (e.g., cross the right arm to pick up the exercise band on the left side of your butt) so that the exercise band crosses over your torso, holding the exercise band with the palm facing up. Rest the other hand on your knee. **INHALE TO BEGIN**.

1 EXHALE: Keep your right elbow glued to your side as you externally rotate your arm to the right, keeping a 90-degree angle at the elbow.

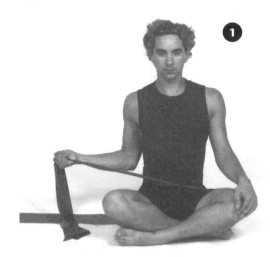

1

BENEFITS	DOS & DON'TS	IMAGINE
■ Strengthens the rotator cuff of the shoulder, specifically the infraspinatus and teres minor. ■ Stretches and rotates the spine.	■ Do keep the neck long in its axis on the spine. ■ Do keep the elbow glued to your side.	■ You are spiraling toward the center of the earth.

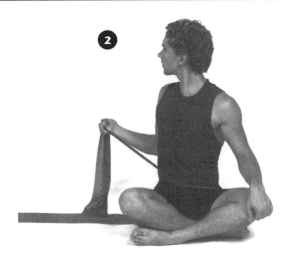

2 Twist the spine toward the right, allowing your head to be the last thing to turn as you spiral. Think "arm, torso, head" when sequencing the spiral open. **INHALE**: Hold, sitting up tall.

3–4 **EXHALE AND INHALE**: Return to the starting position, again sequencing the spiral "arm, torso, head."

repeat	3 times each side

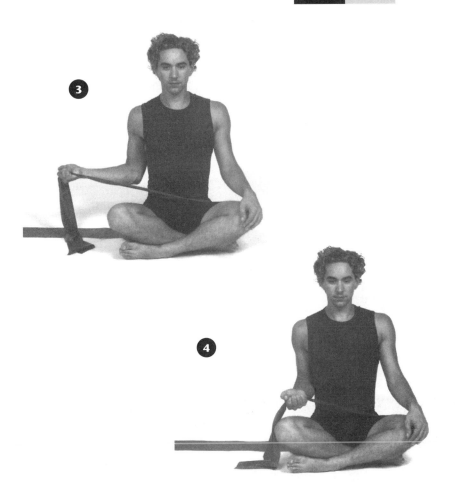

doggie kick

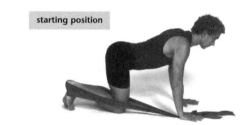

starting position

STARTING POSITION: Start on your hands and knees. Lift one foot slightly off the floor and loop the exercise band around the heel of that foot. Hold the ends down with the same-side arm. **INHALE TO BEGIN**.

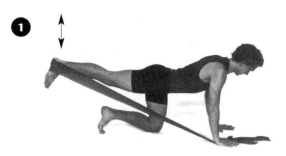

1   ↕

1 **EXHALE**: Extend the leg with the exercise band straight back, pressing through the heel and engaging the buttocks. For additional butt work, pulse up 10 times at this point.

INHALE and retrograde the movement back to starting position.

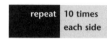

repeat	10 times each side

FTD florist

starting position

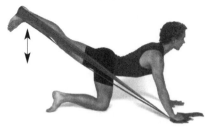

STARTING POSITION: Start on your hands and knees, your back in a C-curve. Lift one foot slightly off the floor and loop the exercise band around the heel of that foot. Hold the ends down with the same-side arm. **INHALE TO BEGIN**.

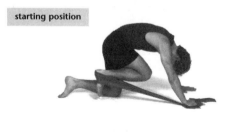

↕

1 **EXHALE**: Extend the leg with the band diagonally back and up, pressing through the heel and engaging the buttocks.

INHALE and retrograde the movement back to starting position.

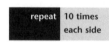

repeat	10 times each side

BENEFITS	DOS & DON'TS	IMAGINE
■ Strengthens the butt and hamstrings.	■ Keep the shoulders relaxed and pulling down the back. ■ Keep the belly scooped. ■ Reach the leg high enough behind you to feel your butt work.	■ You are a doggie at a fire hydrant.

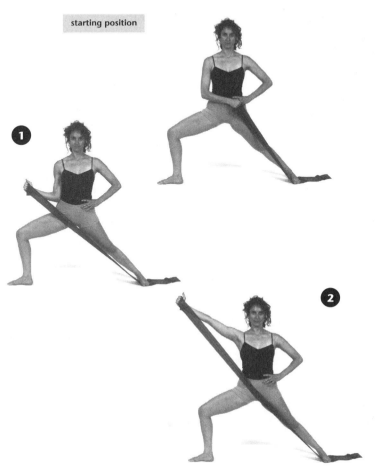

starting position

1

2

STARTING POSITION: Step on one end of the exercise band and hold on to the other end with one hand. Step into a lunge: internally rotate the straight leg and externally rotate the bent knee, keeping the knee aligned over the second toe. This is a "warrior II" position in yoga. **INHALE TO BEGIN**.

1 **EXHALE**: Keeping the elbow glued to the side of the body, externally rotate the arm as far as you can. **INHALE AND HOLD**.

2 **EXHALE:** "Punch" the arm diagonally to the side and slightly in front of the body.

INHALE and retrograde the movement back to the starting position.

repeat	8 times each side

exercise band

VARIATION

This is the more classic Pilates Swackadee from the kneeling side arm series on the Reformer. Begin the same as above, but keep the elbow out to the side of the body and extend the arm diagonally, thinking "elbow-wrist-hand" as you extend. Retrograde the movement, thinking "hand-wrist-elbow" as you return to starting position.

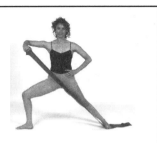

BENEFITS	DOS & DON'TS	IMAGINE
■ Strengthens and stabilizes the shoulders, especially the infraspinatus and teres minor. ■ Opens the chest. ■ Strengthens the legs and butt. ■ Reverses rounded shoulders.	■ Do keep your elbow glued in toward your side and make sure to externally rotate the shoulder as much as possible before punching out.	■ You are saluting the Pilates Goddess.

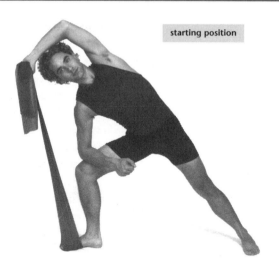

starting position

STARTING POSITION: Stand in a side lunge, keeping the hip bones facing forward; internally rotate the straight leg and externally rotate the bent knee, keeping the knees aligned over the second toes. This is a "warrior II" position in yoga. Stand on the exercise band with the bent knee. Side-bend your torso over the lunging leg and hold the other end of the exercise band with the high hand. Bend the elbow up to the sky with palm facing up. **INHALE TO BEGIN**.

1 **EXHALE**: Keeping the elbow stable and the shoulder down away from the ear, stretch the exercise band up toward the sky.

INHALE and return to starting position.

repeat	8 times each side

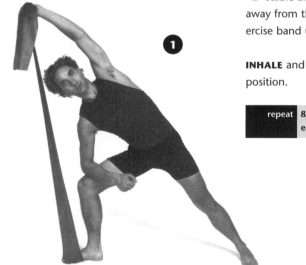

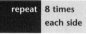

BENEFITS	DOS & DON'TS	IMAGINE
■ Strengthens and stretches the shoulders. ■ Strengthens the legs and butt. ■ Stretches the side of the body.	■ Do keep the working shoulder down away from the ear. ■ Do keep the neck relaxed. ■ Don't let your lunging knee internally rotate; keep the knee aligned over your second toe.	■ You are painting underneath the stairs.

lunging triceps — *beginning*

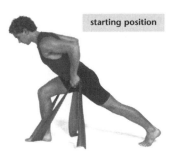

starting position

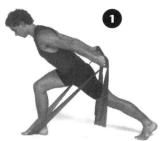

STARTING POSITION: Stand in a lunge with the front leg bent to a 90-degree angle and the back leg lengthened behind you, heel lifted. Stand on the middle of the exercise band with the front foot and hold the ends in each hand. For Lunging Triceps, keep your elbows glued to the sides of your body, arms at a 90-degree angle. **INHALE TO BEGIN**.

1 EXHALE: Extend the arms straight behind you, keeping the elbows pulled into your sides.

INHALE and return to starting position.

repeat	10 times each leg

lunging biceps — *beginning*

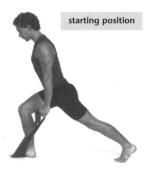

starting position

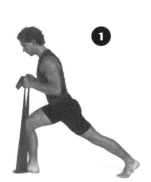

STARTING POSITION: Start in the lunge, holding the band so that the ends come out the thumb side of your fists, arms straight down. **INHALE TO BEGIN**.

1 EXHALE: Pull the exercise band toward your shoulders, bending the elbows as far as you can.

INHALE and return to starting position.

repeat	10 times each leg

BENEFITS	DOS & DON'TS	IMAGINE
■ Strengthens the triceps, quadriceps, glutes, and hamstrings. ■ Stretches the hip flexors.	■ Keep your elbows glued to your body. ■ Keep your lunge aligned with the front knee aligned over the second toe of your front foot.	■ You will no longer have that dingle-dangle under your arm.

lunging series

lunging rhomboids

exercise band

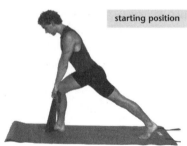

starting position

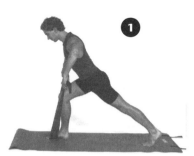

1

STARTING POSITION: Start in the lunge, elbows open and arms straight down. Hold the band so that the ends come out the pinkie side of your fists. **INHALE TO BEGIN**.

1 EXHALE: With your arms straight down, pull the elbows open and wide to the side so that your arms make a square shape with a 90-degree angle at the elbow.

INHALE and return to starting position.

repeat	10 times each leg

lunging chest expansion

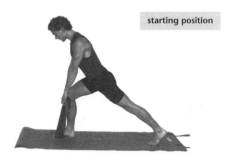

starting position

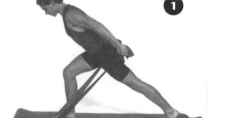

1

STARTING POSITION: Start in the lunge, elbows open and arms straight down. Hold the band so that the ends come out the pinkie side of your fists. **INHALE TO BEGIN**.

1 EXHALE: Pull the arms straight back so they come slightly behind the body.

INHALE and return to starting position.

repeat	10 times each leg

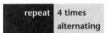

starting position

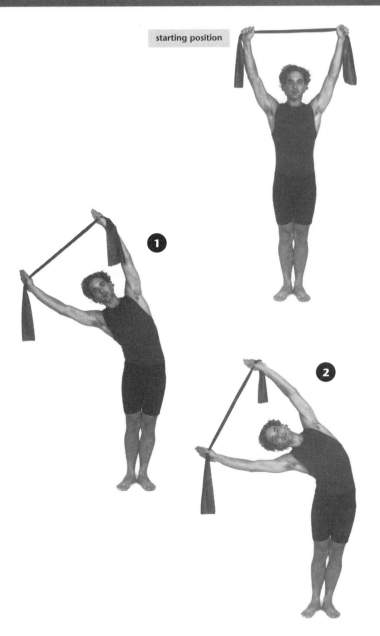

1 **2**

STARTING POSITION: From standing, hold the exercise band overhead. The arms should be shoulder distance apart with some mild tension on the band. **INHALE TO BEGIN**.

1–2 **EXHALE**: Scoop you belly in and lift "up and over a barrel," reaching your arms and torso to one side, arcing your body in a side-bend. Ground the opposite leg to create stretch and stability. **INHALE AND EXHALE**: Hold for one full breath.

INHALE and return to starting position.

repeat	4 times alternating

BENEFITS	DOS & DON'TS	IMAGINE
■ Stretches the side: obliques, quadratus lumborum (QL for short), and lats.	■ Do keep yourself in a two-dimensional plane. ■ Don't arch your back; keep your belly scooped and your buttocks toned.	■ You are a half moon.

exercise band

starting position

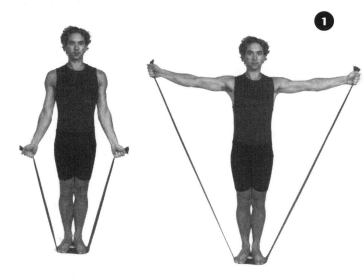

1

STARTING POSITION: Stand on the middle of the exercise band in Pilates First Position, feet slightly turned out from the top of the hip, toes apart, heels together, inner thighs pulling together. Hold on to the ends of the exercise band, one in each hand, thumbs facing up, with a slight bit of tension in the band. **INHALE TO BEGIN**.

1 **EXHALE**: Scoop the belly in and let the shoulders drop down away from the ears as you pull the exercise band up to the sides, making a T shape.

INHALE and return to starting position.

repeat **10 times**

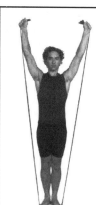

VARIATIONS

If you can keep your shoulders down away from your ears, keep raising your arms like an angel.

For more supraspinatus work, try the same exercise with the thumbs facing down so that the arms are internally rotated. Don't lift your arms higher than 90 degrees in this position.

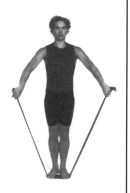

BENEFITS	DOS & DON'TS	IMAGINE
■ Strengthens the supraspinatus muscle. ■ Teaches proper scapular movement.	■ Don't let your shoulders rise up at any point. ■ Keep the neck relaxed.	■ You are one of Charlie's Angels.

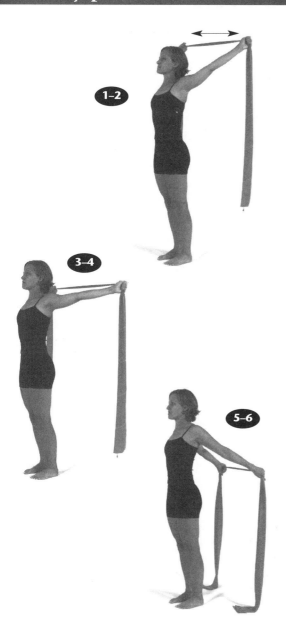

STARTING POSITION: From standing, hold the exercise band behind your torso, with one end in each hand. Begin with your arms diagonally reaching back above your head, elbows facing each other, palms facing away from each other.

1–2 **INHALE**: Open your arms against the resistance. **EXHALE**: Let the exercise band pull the arms closer together behind you. Hold for one full breath, allowing the chest to expand and open forward. Think of squeezing your scapulas together behind you.

3–4 **INHALE**: Open your arms against the resistance and lower them straight back behind you so that they are in line with your armpits. **EXHALE**: Let the exercise band pull the arms closer together behind you. Hold for one full breath, allowing the chest to expand and open forward. Think of squeezing your scapulas together behind you.

5–6 **INHALE**: Open your arms against the resistance and lower them slightly. Internally rotate the arms, turning the elbows out and the palms toward each other. **EXHALE**: Let the exercise band pull the arms closer together behind you. Hold for one full breath, allowing the chest to expand and open forward. Think of squeezing your scapulas together behind you.

repeat | once

BENEFITS	DOS & DON'TS	IMAGINE
■ Stretches the chest and pectoral muscles. ■ Activates the upper back muscles.	■ Do stick your chest out and lean into the stretch. ■ Do inhale deeply and allow the intercostal spaces to expand.	■ You are Kate Winslet suspended off the front of the *Titanic*.

exercise band

rotator strengthener

beginning

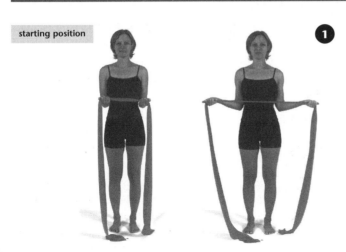

starting position

1

STARTING POSITION: Stand holding the band from underneath, elbows glued to your sides, fists facing up. **INHALE TO BEGIN**.

1 EXHALE: Keeping your elbows in by your sides, rotate your arms open to the sides. Make sure your elbows don't slide backward. Hold for one full breath.

INHALE and control back to the starting position.

repeat **10 times**

rhomboids strengthener

beginning

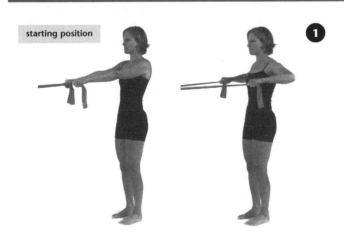

starting position

1

STARTING POSITION: Wrap the exercise band around something stable that is approximately the height of your shoulders; hold on to each end. **INHALE TO BEGIN**.

1 EXHALE: Keep your shoulders pulling down your back as you pull your elbows back, keeping a square shape in your elbows. Reach back behind your body until you feel your back muscles engaging. Hold for one full breath.

INHALE and return to starting position.

repeat **10 times**

BENEFITS	DOS & DON'TS
■ Strengthens and stabilizes the shoulder muscles. ■ Opens the chest. ■ Reverses rounded shoulders.	■ Don't let your shoulders creep up. ■ Keep the neck long and relaxed.

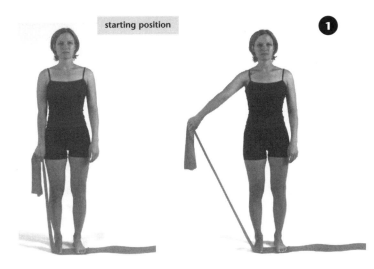

starting position

STARTING POSITION: Stand with your back to a wall, knees soft, chest and shoulders open and keeping contact with the wall. Step on one end of the exercise band with one foot and hold the other end with the same-side hand; keep the arm internally rotated, thumb down to the floor. Make sure the exercise band is pulled taut enough so that there is already resistance when the hand is down by the side of the body. **INHALE TO BEGIN**.

1 EXHALE: Keeping your shoulders pulling down your back, slowly raise the exercise band to the side and slightly in front of you. Do not raise the arm higher than 90 degrees. Hold for one full breath.

repeat	10 times each side

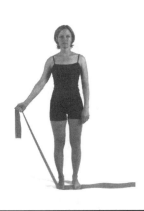

VARIATION

Pulsing Variation: Start in the same position except turn the working arm so that the shoulder is externally rotated with the thumb facing up. Make sure the exercise band has tension at the start of the exercise. Then pulse the arm straight up to the side (pure abduction), keeping your shoulders down your back. Repeat 30 times fast.

BENEFITS	DOS & DON'TS	IMAGINE
■ Strengthens and stabilizes the shoulder, especially the supraspinatus.	■ Do keep the range of motion of the shoulder small; the supraspinatus only works in the first 15–20 degrees of abduction.	■ You are pouring out a can of beer (keeping very good alignment all the while!).

starting position

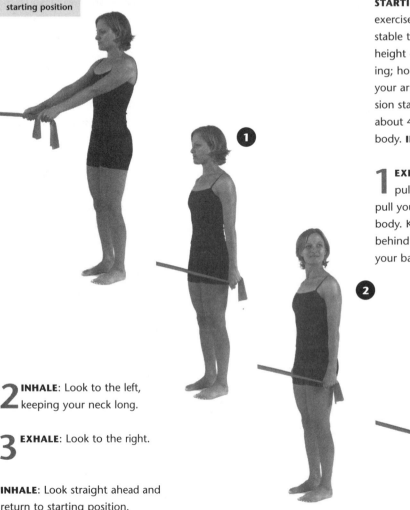

STARTING POSITION: Wrap the exercise band around something stable that is approximately the height of your hands when standing; hold on to each end, keeping your arms straight, with the tension starting when the arms are about 45 degrees in front of the body. **INHALE TO BEGIN.**

1 EXHALE: Keep your shoulders pulling down your back as you pull your arms to the sides of your body. Keep pulling back slightly behind your body until you feel your back muscles engaging.

2 INHALE: Look to the left, keeping your neck long.

3 EXHALE: Look to the right.

INHALE: Look straight ahead and return to starting position.

repeat 10 times

BENEFITS	DOS & DON'TS
■ Strengthens and stabilizes the shoulders, especially the lats, rhomboids, mid traps, infraspinatus, and teres minor. ■ Opens the chest. ■ Good for thoracic outlet syndrome. ■ Reverses rounded shoulders.	■ Don't let your shoulders creep up. ■ Keep the neck long and relaxed.

starting position

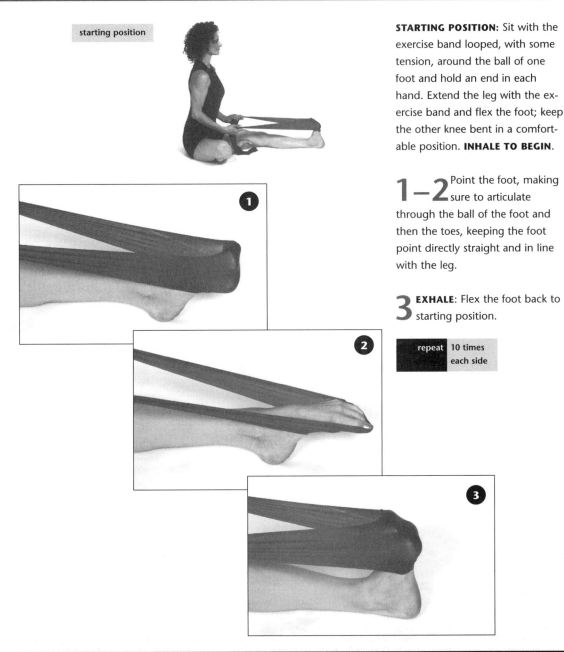

STARTING POSITION: Sit with the exercise band looped, with some tension, around the ball of one foot and hold an end in each hand. Extend the leg with the exercise band and flex the foot; keep the other knee bent in a comfortable position. **INHALE TO BEGIN.**

1–2 Point the foot, making sure to articulate through the ball of the foot and then the toes, keeping the foot point directly straight and in line with the leg.

3 **EXHALE:** Flex the foot back to starting position.

repeat | 10 times each side

exercise band

BENEFITS	DOS & DON'TS	IMAGINE
■ Strengthens the intrinsic muscles of the foot, arch, and calf. ■ Strengthens the ankle. ■ Teaches proper foot and ankle alignment.	■ Do keep the foot pointing straight ahead. ■ Don't let the foot make an arc as it points and flexes; think of it staying in its narrow track.	■ You are a ballet dancer warming up for *Swan Lake*.

exercise band

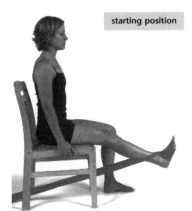

starting position

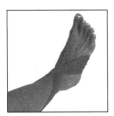

1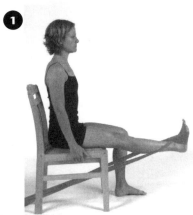

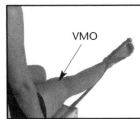

VMO

VARIATION

Try the same exercise with slight external rotation to help get the VMO firing.

STARTING POSITION: Sit on a chair and tie the exercise band around the back leg of the chair or to something stable behind you at approximately the height of your ankle. Wrap the front loop of the exercise band like a sandal around your foot: first twist the loop once, then place your toes into the front of the loop. This exercise can be done in shoes, too. **INHALE TO BEGIN:** Sit up tall and lift your foot so that there is some tension in the band, knee bent only about 15–20 degrees.

1 EXHALE: Extend your knee all the way, making sure to fire the VMO (vastus medialis obliquus), the most medial fibers of your quadriceps that fire on the last few degrees of extension. Hold for one full breath.

INHALE and return to starting position, again bending the knee only about 15–20 degrees.

repeat **10 times each side**

BENEFITS	DOS & DON'TS	IMAGINE
▪ Strengthens the quads, especially the VMO. ▪ Helps stabilize the knee after injury. ▪ Can correct patellar tracking problems.	▪ Do make sure to hold the extension and make that VMO tremble! ▪ Don't bend the knee more than 20 degrees. ▪ Do keep the thigh as relaxed as possible on the chair; try not to grip at the hip.	▪ You are pulling your knee cap toward your inner thigh as you extend the knee.

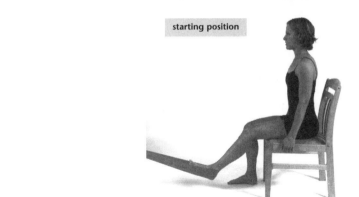

starting position

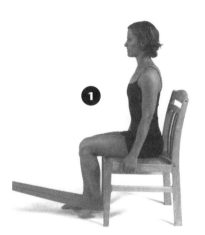

1

STARTING POSITION: Sit on a chair and tie the exercise band around something stable in front of you (like the leg of a heavy table or bureau) that's at the height of your ankle. Place one foot inside the free loop, making sure the exercise band is spread evenly around the heel. Pull the chair back so that you feel some resistance when you start the exercise; your leg should start at about 135 degrees of extension. **INHALE TO BEGIN**: Sit up tall.

1 **EXHALE:** Pull the heel back against the resistance as far as the chair allows, keeping your heel aligned straight under your thigh.

INHALE and return to starting position, keeping some tension in the exercise band.

repeat	10 times each side

BENEFITS	DOS & DON'TS	IMAGINE
■ Strengthens the hamstrings. ■ Helps stabilize the knee after injury, especially after an ACL (anterior cruciate ligament) tear.	■ Do keep the thigh as relaxed as possible on the chair; try not to grip at the hip. ■ Do make sure that you have some resistance when you begin so that by the time your knee is at 90 degrees, you have really worked that hamstring.	■ You will be out on the dance floor soon.

starting position

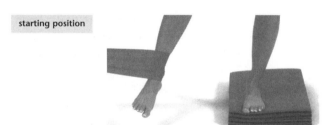

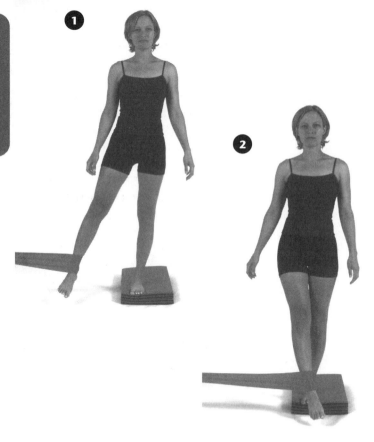

STARTING POSITION: Tie the exercise band to something stable that's at your ankle height (the leg of a heavy table or bureau). Put your foot inside the exercise band so that the loop wraps around the inner ankle of the leg closest to the exercise band. Stand far enough away to feel tension in the exercise band with the leg straight and held out to the side approximately 45 degrees from the centerline. You can stand on something or wear a shoe on the standing leg to raise yourself up a little; this helps clear the working leg.

1 **INHALE TO BEGIN:** Stand tall on your supporting leg, pulling your belly in.

2 **EXHALE:** Pull the extended leg in toward the centerline, thinking of lengthening through the heel, and keep pulling until your leg crosses the other.

repeat	10 times each side

BENEFITS	**DOS & DON'TS**	**IMAGINE**
■ Strengthens the adductors (inner thigh muscles) of the leg. ■ Helps stabilize the knee after injury. The standing leg also gets a great stabilization challenge.	■ Do stand tall and in parallel, keeping the standing leg grounded through the inner thigh.	■ You are actually working the standing leg as much as the moving leg.

starting position

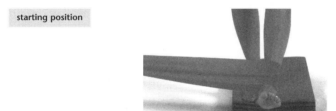

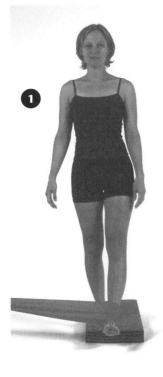

1

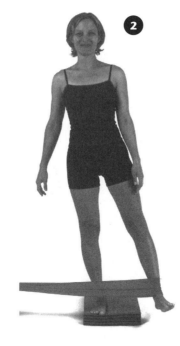

2

STARTING POSITION: Tie the exercise band to something stable that's at your ankle height (the leg of a heavy table or bureau). Put your foot inside the exercise band so that the loop wraps around the outside ankle of the leg which is further from the exercise band. The standing leg should be slightly behind the working leg so that the exercise band clears the front of the body. Stand far enough away to feel tension in the exercise band with the leg straight and slightly pulled across your centerline. You can stand on something or wear a shoe on the standing leg to raise yourself up a little; this helps clear the working leg.

1 **INHALE TO BEGIN:** Stand tall on your supporting leg, pulling your belly in.

2 **EXHALE:** Pull the working leg to the side approximately 45 degrees from the centerline. Think of lengthening through the heel of the working leg.

repeat	10 times each side

BENEFITS	DOS & DON'TS	IMAGINE
■ Strengthens the abductors (outer thigh muscles) of the leg and hip, specifically the gluteus medius and TFL (tensor fasciae latae) of the working leg. ■ Helps stabilize the knee after injury. The standing leg also gets a great stabilization challenge.	■ Do stand tall and in parallel, keeping the standing leg grounded through the inner thigh.	■ You are standing tall on one leg.

3-way hip stretch

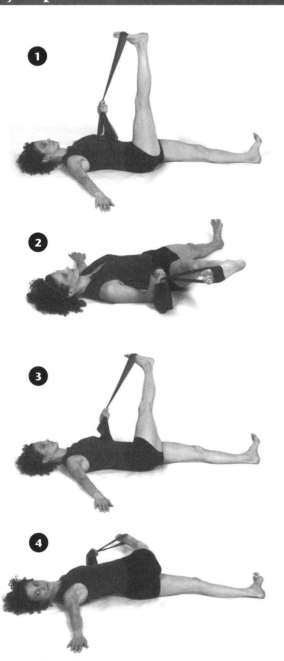

STARTING POSITION: Lie on your back with the exercise band looped around one foot and reach that leg up to the sky. Extend the other leg down on the mat in front of you. **INHALE AND EXHALE CONTINUOUSLY:**

1 *Hamstring:* Pull the leg toward your body, keeping the knee straight. If you have very tight hamstrings, you'll have to use your quadriceps to keep the knee straight. Try to ground your tailbone to increase the stretch.

2 *Adductor:* Put the exercise band in the same hand as the stretching leg and open the leg out to the side, externally rotating the leg from the hip. Try to ground your tailbone to increase the stretch.

3 *Abductor:* Hold the exercise band in the opposite hand of the stretching leg and let the leg internally rotate from the hip and slowly cross over your body. Try to ground your tailbone to increase the stretch.

4 *Spine Twist:* Keep crossing the leg until it reaches the floor.

repeat	once each side

BENEFITS	DOS & DON'TS	IMAGINE
■ Stretches the muscles of the hip.	■ Do breathe to help elongate the muscles. ■ Don't allow tension to creep up into the neck and shoulders.	■ You will have open hips some day.

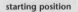
starting position

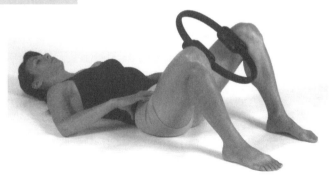

STARTING POSITION: Lie on your back, knees bent with the magic circle (or small ball) between your knees, feet flat on the floor, hip distance apart. Place your hands on your low abdomen, right inside your hip bones (the anterior superior iliac spine, or ASIS). **INHALE TO BEGIN**.

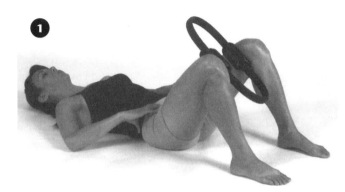

1 EXHALE: During the first half of your exhale, simply let your abdominals melt down into your spine. Then, keeping your abs as scooped as possible, squeeze your circle, imagining the initiation of the squeeze coming from the abdominals under your fingers. You should feel the muscles under your fingers hardening as you squeeze the circle. You are pulling your hip bones toward each other with your abdominals as you squeeze your circle.

INHALE and return to starting position, allowing the circle to slowly release.

repeat **5 times**

circle/small ball

BENEFITS	DOS & DON'TS	IMAGINE
■ Strengthens the inner thighs. ■ Teaches the deep abdominal scoop and the synergistic connection between the oblique abdominals and the inner thighs.	■ Do release the circle on the inhale—give those inner thighs a rest! ■ Keep neutral spine when scooping and squeezing; it's easy to tuck under during this part.	■ Your legs originate from your belly.

upper abdominal curls *beginning*

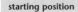
starting position

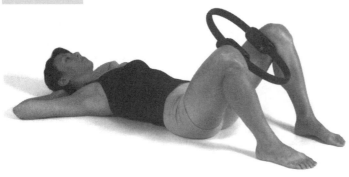

STARTING POSITION: Lie on your back with your knees bent, feet flat on the floor, hip distance apart. Hold the magic circle (or small ball) between your knees. Interlace your fingers behind your head, elbows wide. **INHALE TO BEGIN. EXHALE**: Begin with the deep abdominal cue (see previous page), scooping your belly in as you squeeze the circle on the first half of your exhale.

1 On the second half of the exhale, Squeeze a Tangerine under your chin as you lift your head off the mat and roll up to the Pilates Abdominal Positioning. Anchor your sternum to the mat and think of lengthening your spine as you roll up. **INHALE**: Hold.

EXHALE and return to starting position.

1

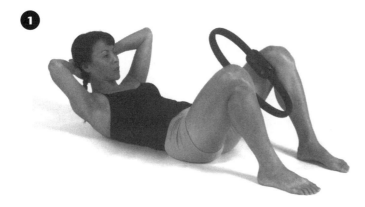

| repeat | 5 times |

BENEFITS	DOS & DON'TS	IMAGINE
■ Strengthens the inner thighs, abdominals, and neck flexors. ■ Stretches the back of the neck and upper back.	■ Do maintain neutral spine when rolling up. ■ Don't let your low back flatten.	■ You are stretching your upper back as you roll up.

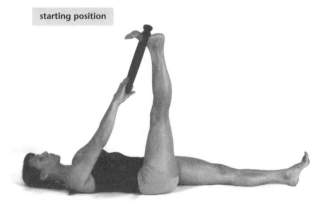

starting position

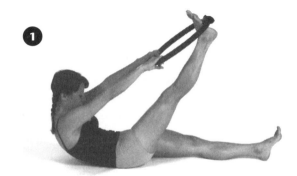

1

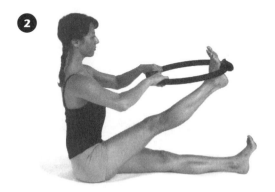

2

STARTING POSITION: Lie on your back. Hold the magic circle with both hands and place your foot inside the circle. Both legs are straight, one along the floor, the other inside the circle reaching up toward the sky. Keep your elbows slightly bent and open to the sides, neck relaxed and shoulders down the back. **INHALE TO BEGIN**.

1 Scoop your belly in toward your spine as you reach away with the heel in the circle and begin to roll up off the mat, Squeezing a Tangerine under your chin and articulating through the spine.

2 **INHALE**: Stack up from the base of your spine, keeping your leg in the circle as high as possible.

EXHALE: Pull the navel in toward your spine and press away with your heel as you roll back down, one vertebra at a time. Return to starting position.

repeat	4 times each side

BENEFITS	DOS & DON'TS
■ Strengthens the abdominals and hip flexors. ■ Creates articulation in the spine. ■ Stretches the hamstrings.	■ Do use the energy through the reaching leg to help you roll up. ■ Don't tense your upper body; keep the neck relaxed and elbows wide.

circle/small ball

starting position

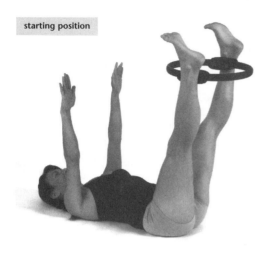

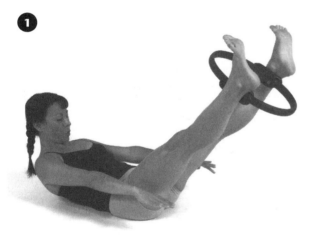

1

STARTING POSITION: Lie on your back with your arms and legs reaching up to the sky, palms facing forward. Hold the magic circle (or small ball) between your ankles. **INHALE TO BEGIN**.

1 **EXHALE**: Roll up to the Pilates Abdominal Positioning, reaching your arms toward the floor as you diagonally extend your legs away from the body. The lower the legs, the more abdominal challenge. Begin a percussive beating of the arms, small and controlled, a few inches from the floor. **INHALE** through your nose, counting out 5 beats with your arms, and then **EXHALE** through your mouth, making a shushing sound on every beat for 5 beats...until you count to 100 beats of your arms. Maintain your abdominal positioning the whole time.

repeat	10 breaths
	x 10 beats
	= 100 counts

BENEFITS

- Strengthens the deep neck flexors, abdominals, and hip flexors.
- Stabilizes the lower back.
- Helps you practice percussive breathing.

DOS & DON'TS

- Make sure to keep the Abdominal Scoop.
- Maintain a flat back by scooping the belly in toward the spine; don't let the back arch off the floor.
- Don't let your upper body roll down from the abdominal positioning; on every exhale make sure your shoulder blades are just off the floor.
- Feel the arms pulsing from the back (latissimus dorsi) rather than from the pectorals.

- Avoid if you have an acute neck injury. This exercise can be hard on the neck, especially if the back of your neck (trapezius muscle) is tight.
- If you have a tight upper back, it may be difficult for you to maintain your upper abdominal curl. Just keep trying!

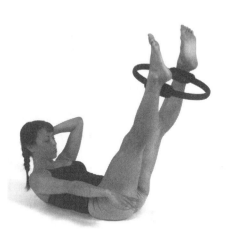

MODIFICATION

Put one hand behind your head to support your neck if you feel strain.

VARIATIONS

Hundred *beginning*

Keep knees bent in Table Top Position and put the circle between your knees.

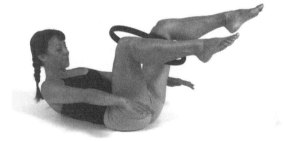

Hundred *advanced*

Lower your legs as far as you can while still maintaining a flat low back on the mat.

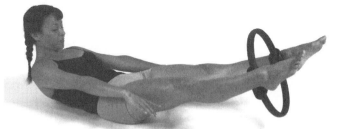

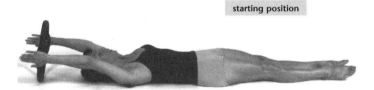

circle/small ball

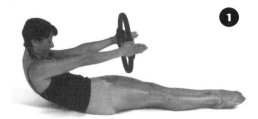

starting position

STARTING POSITION: Lie on your back with the magic circle (or small ball) in your hands reaching up by your ears. Extend your legs straight down on the floor, inner thighs squeezing together in Pilates First Position (slightly turned out). **INHALE TO BEGIN**.

1 **EXHALE**: Lift the circle up and forward as you roll up, Squeezing a Tangerine under your chin as you sequence the spine off the floor, and squeezing your inner thighs and buns together to assist you in the roll-up.

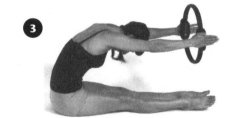

3 Finish with a C-curve of your whole spine, circle reaching forward. **INHALE**: Hold the stretch.

EXHALE: Retrograde the movement until you're down on your back. **INHALE** to reach your arms by your ears, flowing right through to step 1.

repeat **4 times**

VARIATIONS

beginner

To make the roll-up easier, bend your knees and press your feet into the floor.

advanced

To make the roll-up more difficult, keep the circle by your ears the whole time.

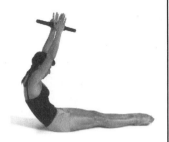

BENEFITS

- Strengthens the abdominals and hip flexors.
- Creates articulation in the spine.

DOS & DON'TS

- Don't let your feet come up off the floor; bend your knees if you need to.
- Weak abdominals and hip flexors will make this exercise not only difficult but dangerous for your lower back. Make sure you can do this exercise without the circle before attempting it with the extra load.

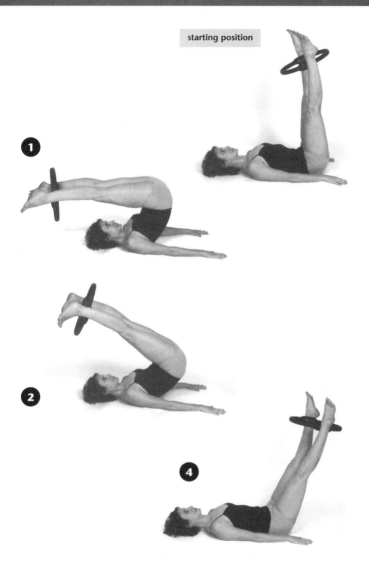

starting position

STARTING POSITION: Lie on your back with your legs straight up toward the sky, magic circle (or small ball) between your ankles and Door Frame Arms down by your sides, palms facing down. **INHALE TO BEGIN**.

1 **EXHALE**: Scoop your belly in as you lift the circle up and over your head. Reach the circle to the wall behind you, with your weight balanced between your shoulder blades. Press your arms down onto the floor to help control the movement.

2 **INHALE**: Flex your feet, then **EXHALE** and roll down your spine, one vertebra at a time, reaching long through your heels. Control the movement with your Abdominal Scoop until your hips reach down to the floor.

4 **INHALE**: Keep the belly scooped and the low back flat as you drop your legs to the diagonal.

repeat **4 times**

BENEFITS	DOS & DON'TS	
* Stretches and articulates the spine. * Strengthens the abdominals, inner thighs, triceps, and lats.	■ Press the arms down to control your movements, but don't let the shoulders hunch up by your ears—keep them stabilized down the back.	■ Don't roll onto your neck. ■ Try to articulate through each vertebra by pulling your belly in and pressing the low back onto the floor as you roll back.

starting position

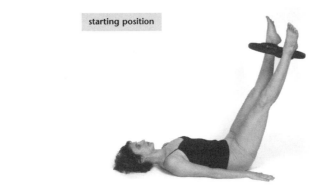

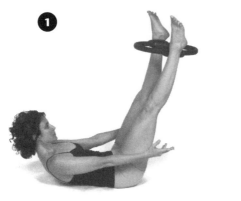

1

2

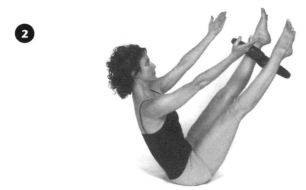

STARTING POSITION: Lie on your back with the magic circle or small ball between your ankles, reaching the legs up diagonally, arms down by your sides, palms facing up. Your belly is scooped in and your low back is flat on the floor. **INHALE TO BEGIN**.

1 **EXHALE**: Squeeze a Tangerine under your chin as you lift your head off the floor, pulling your shoulder blades down your back as you reach forward with your arms. Scoop your belly in and squeeze the circle and your butt as you roll all the way up to your balance point, stopping just before you reach your tailbone.

2 At the top of the Teaser, reach your arms up and forward as you try to lift your chest while keeping your low belly scooped in. **INHALE** at the top.

EXHALE: Scoop your belly in and squeeze your circle as you roll all the way down your spine, allowing your arms to trail down to the starting position.

| repeat | 4 times |

BENEFITS	**DOS & DON'TS**	**IMAGINE**
■ Strengthens the abdominals and hip flexors. ■ Articulates the spine.	■ Tight hamstrings will make this exercise much more difficult; if you suffer from this, do the Diamond-leg or Bent-knee variations. ■ Make sure to keep the shoulders down away from the ears.	■ An energy force pulls the shoulder blades down the back as you initiate the roll up into your Teaser, then travels down and around to the front as you scoop your belly in. Back to front. We call this the Serrape.

VARIATIONS

Bent-knee Teaser
intermediate

Bend the knees, keeping them parallel.

Diamond-leg Teaser
intermediate

Perform the Teaser with the knees open to a diamond shape, the circle between the ankles.

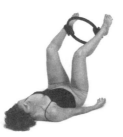
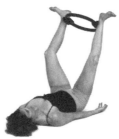

Dead-hang Teaser   *super-advanced*

With your legs lengthened out in front of you, just off the mat, and your arms extended back by your ears, fold your body into Teaser. Inhale and unfold your body, keeping your arms by your ears as you lower your legs and upper body down toward the floor. Come down into a "dead hang." Repeat Teaser to dead hang 3 times.

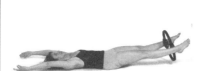
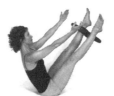
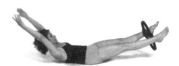

"dead hang"

Teaser into Open-leg Rocker   *super-advanced*

Roll up into the Teaser position and grab onto your calves. Repeat 3 times and then finish with the Open-leg Rocker 3 times.

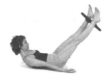

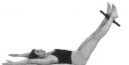

circle/small ball

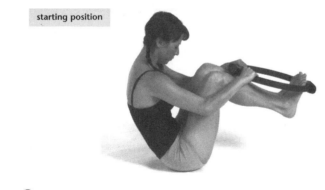

starting position

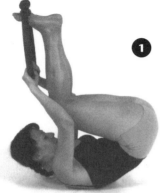

1

STARTING POSITION: Sit up and put your feet inside the magic circle, holding on to the other side. Bend your knees in toward your chest and squeeze your knees and inner thighs together. Your elbows are bent and open to the sides, your neck is relaxed, and your shoulders are pulled down your back. You should be in your Balance Point, sitting just behind your tailbone, low belly scooped in and low back slightly rounded. **INHALE TO BEGIN**.

1 EXHALE: Roll back onto your shoulder blades, articulating through your spine. Think of pressing through your feet to engage the backs of your legs.

INHALE and roll back to your Balance Point.

repeat **5 times**

VARIATION

intermediate

To increase the difficulty, place your hands in front of the knees and the magic circle between the ankles.

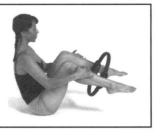

BENEFITS	DOS & DON'TS	IMAGINE
■ Stretches and articulates the spine. ■ Strengthens the abdominals, hamstrings, and inner thighs.	■ Don't do if you have a neck injury. ■ Don't roll onto your neck; instead, balance between your shoulder blades. See "How to Do a Rolling Exercise" on page 13 for further instructions on how to avoid neck problems. ■ Don't "thump." If your low back is tight, you will have difficulty rolling smoothly over that area. Slow down and use your Abdominal Scoop to get the low back pressing onto the floor.	■ You are massaging your spine as you roll, trying to get every vertebra in contact with the floor.

straight-leg rocker · *advanced*

starting position

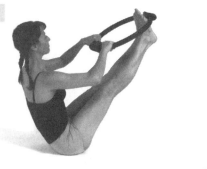

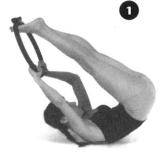

1

STARTING POSITION: Sit up and put your feet inside the magic circle, holding on to the other side. Extend your legs out, keeping your legs squeezed together. Your elbows are bent and open to the sides, your neck is relaxed, and your shoulders are pulled down your back. You should be in your Balance Point. **INHALE TO BEGIN**.

1 **EXHALE**: Roll back onto your shoulder blades, articulating through your spine. Think of pressing through your feet to engage the backs of your legs.

INHALE and roll back to your Balance Point.

repeat 5 times

open-leg rocker · *advanced*

starting position

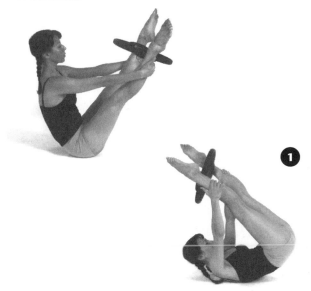

1

STARTING POSITION: Sit up and hold the magic circle between your ankles. Grab onto your calves and extend your legs out. Your neck is relaxed and your shoulders are pulled down your back. You should be in your Balance Point. **INHALE TO BEGIN**.

1 **EXHALE**: Roll back onto your shoulder blades, articulating through your spine. Think of pressing through your feet to engage the backs of your legs.

INHALE and roll back to your Balance Point.

repeat 5 times

circle/small ball

112

classic abs series
single-leg stretch
beginning

starting position

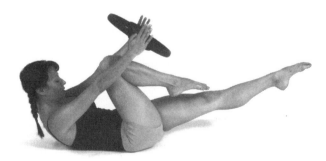

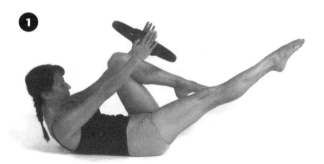

1

This Classic Abs Series is also commonly known as "The Fives."

STARTING POSITION: Start on your back with your right knee folded into your chest; extend the left leg long on a diagonal. Hold the magic circle or small ball between your hands and reach it up to the sky and forward of your knees with straight arms as you roll up to the Pilates Abdominal Position. Your shoulder blades are just off the floor. **INHALE TO BEGIN**.

1 Switch legs, reaching your right leg long, and pull your left knee into your chest. **EXHALE** and repeat 16 times, alternating 2 leg movements on each inhale and 2 on each exhale.

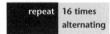

repeat	16 times alternating

BENEFITS	DOS & DON'TS	IMAGINE
■ Strengthens the inner thighs. ■ Teaches the deep abdominal scoop and the synergistic connection between the oblique abdominals and the inner thighs.	■ Do release the circle on the inhale—give those inner thighs a rest! ■ Keep neutral spine when scooping and squeezing; it's easy to tuck under during this part.	■ Your legs originate from your belly.

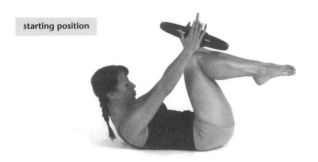

starting position

STARTING POSITION: Lie on your back, knees folded into your chest, and hold the magic circle or small ball, reaching your hands in front of your knees. **INHALE TO BEGIN**.

1 **EXHALE**: Keeping your low back flat on the floor and belly scooped in, lengthen both legs diagonally and reach the circle back by your ears. **INHALE** and return to starting position.

repeat **6 times**

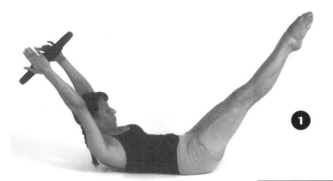

1

circle/small ball

VARIATION

You can also put the magic circle between your ankles. Imagine you're still holding a circle between your hands, and perform the Double-leg Stretch as described above. Do this variation 3 times then the basic move 3 times.

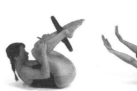
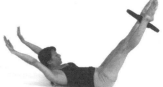

BENEFITS	DOS & DON'TS	
■ Strengthens the neck flexors, abdominals, hip flexors, and lats. ■ Stabilizes the lower back.	■ Don't let your head fall back as you reach your arms by your ears. The only things moving should be your arms and legs! Keep your head perfectly stable by keeping your focus on your belly, not on the moving circle. ■ As in all exercises where your legs are extended to challenge your core, you must monitor yourself to protect your	low back. Only reach your legs as low as you can while still maintaining a flat low back and scooped belly. (See "How to Modify to Protect Your Low Back" on page 13.) ■ Avoid if you have an acute neck injury.

starting position

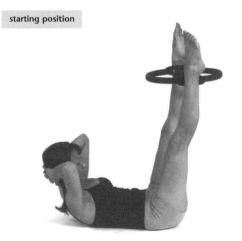

STARTING POSITION: Lie on your back and interlace your fingers behind your head, elbows wide, magic circle between your ankles, legs reaching up to the sky. Keeping your navel scooped in and low back flat on the mat, roll up in the Pilates Abdominal Positioning. **INHALE TO BEGIN**.

1 EXHALE: Keeping your low back flat on the floor and belly scooped in, lower your legs about 12 inches.

INHALE and return to starting position with a perky lift from the belly, accentuating the scoop and the accent on the "up" movement.

repeat 10 times

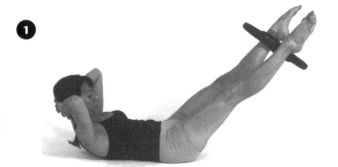

BENEFITS	DOS & DON'TS	IMAGINE
■ Strengthens the neck flexors, abdominals, and hip flexors. ■ Stabilizes the lower back.	■ Don't do if you have an acute neck injury. ■ Do accent the "up" movement of the legs. ■ To protect your low back, only reach your legs as low as you can while still maintaining a flat low back and scooped belly. (See "How to Modify to Protect Your Low Back" on page 13.)	■ Your legs are light as feathers.

VARIATION

Ribcage Control *intermediate*

Start the same as the Double-leg Lowers, except when you roll up to the abdominal positioning to begin, keep the knees bent in toward the chest. Inhale to begin, and on the exhale, keeping your low back flat on the floor and belly scooped in, extend your legs diagonally away from you as you lower your head to the mat. Your head should reach the floor as the legs come to full extension. On the inhale, return to the starting position and try to do a slow-motion hip-up, keeping your belly scooped in.

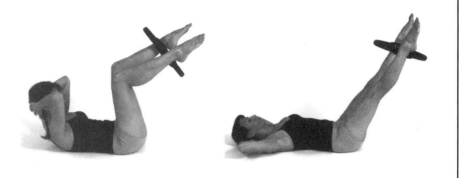

circle/small ball

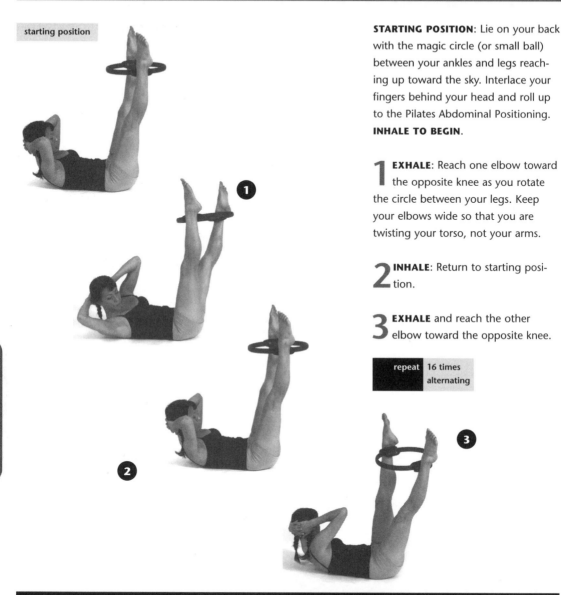

starting position

STARTING POSITION: Lie on your back with the magic circle (or small ball) between your ankles and legs reaching up toward the sky. Interlace your fingers behind your head and roll up to the Pilates Abdominal Positioning. **INHALE TO BEGIN**.

1 **EXHALE**: Reach one elbow toward the opposite knee as you rotate the circle between your legs. Keep your elbows wide so that you are twisting your torso, not your arms.

2 **INHALE**: Return to starting position.

3 **EXHALE** and reach the other elbow toward the opposite knee.

repeat	16 times alternating

BENEFITS	DOS & DON'TS	IMAGINE
■ Strengthens the neck flexors, inner thighs, hip flexors, and abdominals (especially the internal and external obliques).	■ Don't allow your upper body to roll down from the Pilates Abdominal Positioning. Keep the shoulder blades off the floor the whole time. ■ Keep your elbows wide so that you are twisting your torso, not your arms. ■ Think of rotating your trunk from the back, imagining your shoulder blades wrapping around to the front as you twist the upper body.	■ You are rotating around a rotisserie that anchors your sternum to the floor.

starting position

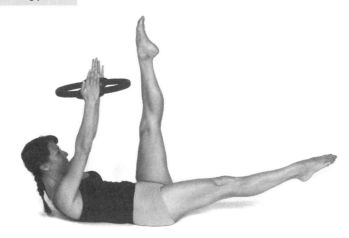

STARTING POSITION: Lie on your back, holding the magic circle in your hands, arms extended up and forward. Extend one leg down, just off the mat; extend the other leg up to the sky. **INHALE TO BEGIN**, gently pulsing the leg toward your nose.

1 **EXHALE**: Switch legs and gently pulse the leg toward your nose.

repeat	20 times alternating

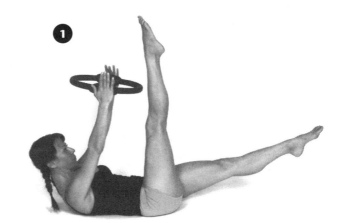

circle/small ball

BENEFITS	DOS & DON'TS
■ Strengthens the neck flexors, abdominals, hip flexors, and lats. ■ Stabilizes the lower back.	■ Keep your legs perfectly straight. If you have tight hamstrings, really use your quads! ■ Avoid if you have an acute neck injury.

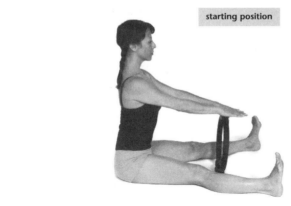

starting position

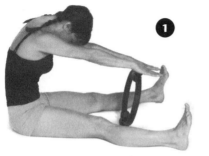

1

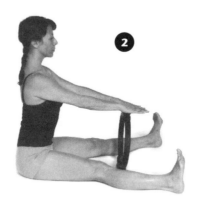

2

STARTING POSITION: Sit up with your legs extended, hip distance apart, feet flexed. Extend your arms forward on top of the magic circle held between your legs. **INHALE TO BEGIN** by lifting your belly up off your hips, and engaging your glutes by pulling your sits bones together.

1 EXHALE: Trying not to lose any height, pull your navel in toward your spine as you round your back up and forward into a C-curve, starting from the base of your spine and sequencing up to your head. Your back should end in the shape of a capital "C." Meanwhile, press down on the magic circle, keeping your shoulders down away from your ears.

2 INHALE: Stack up from the base of your spine, letting your head be the last thing to rise. Sit up tall to start again.

EXHALE: Let the shoulders drop down as you return to starting position.

repeat **3 times**

BENEFITS	DOS & DON'TS	IMAGINE
■ Stretches the whole spine from coccyx to occiput. ■ Creates length in the spine while rounding forward. ■ Allows you to practice the C-curve. ■ Articulates and stacks the spine.	■ Tight hamstrings will limit your ability to sit up straight with your legs straight in front of you. Bend your knees to ease the hamstrings. ■ Don't roll back behind your sits bones; think of staying the same height as you round forward.	■ You must lift up and over a barrel that sits on your lap in order to reach forward.

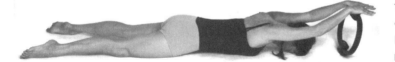

starting position

STARTING POSITION: Lie on your belly with your forehead on the floor, arms up on the magic circle or small ball, legs turned out and hip distance apart. **INHALE TO BEGIN**.

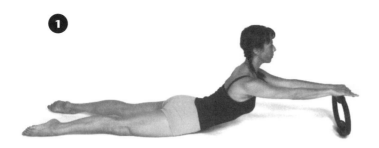

1

1 EXHALE: Pull the shoulders down away from your ears, press down on the circle, then raise your head and upper body up off the floor. Come up to your fullest upper back extension, making sure to protect your lower back by scooping your belly up off the floor, pressing your pubic bone down on the floor, and squeezing your butt.

INHALE and return to the floor.

repeat | 4 times

circle/small ball

BENEFITS	DOS & DON'TS	IMAGINE
■ Strengthens the back and neck extensors. ■ Stretches the lats and pecs.	■ Make sure to keep the shoulders down and the neck long. ■ If you feel compression in your low back, scoop your belly in as much as you can. If you still feel compression, don't come up so high. ■ Don't let your head be a Broken Bud at the top of your spine. The head should always follow the arc of the spine. (See page 19 for further instructions.)	■ As you lift your head, you are watching an ant crawling away from you on the floor. (This image will keep your head and neck on the right track.)

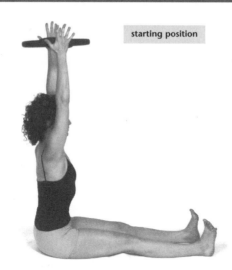

starting position

STARTING POSITION: Sit up with your legs straight in front of you, hip distance apart, feet flexed. With the magic circle or small ball between your hands, reach your arms up to the sky.

1 INHALE: Lift up off your hips and scoop the belly as you hinge back as far as you can, keeping your spine straight.

2 EXHALE: Scoop your belly in. Shovel your pelvis under, creating a C-curve in your low back, and roll down one vertebra at a time, reaching your circle diagonally up and forward.

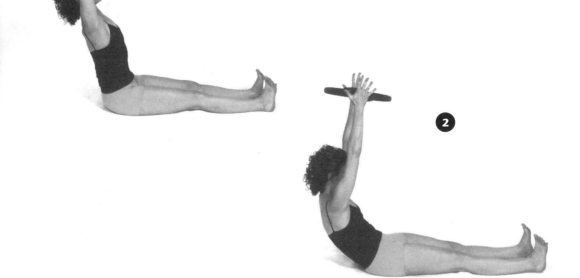

BENEFITS	DOS & DON'TS
■ Strengthens abdominals and hip flexors. ■ Articulates the spine.	■ Activate your legs on the roll down and the roll up by reaching long through your heels. ■ Remember: This is the hardest roll-up!

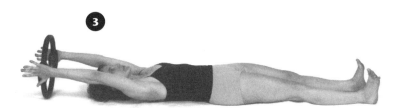

3 INHALE: Finish flat on your back with your arms and the circle reaching back behind you.

4 EXHALE: Lift the circle up to the sky. Squeeze a Tangerine under your chin to lift your head and begin to roll up, reaching the circle up and forward.

5 INHALE: Stack your spine, reaching the circle up to the sky.

repeat | 4 times

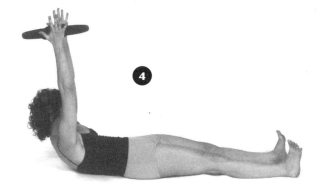

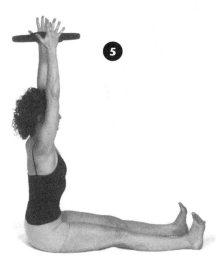

circle/small ball

VARIATION

If you have difficulty articulating into your low back, bend your knees and place your feet on the floor.

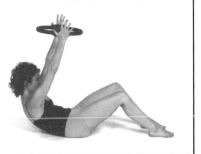

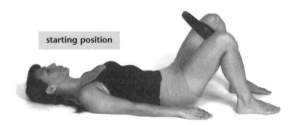

starting position

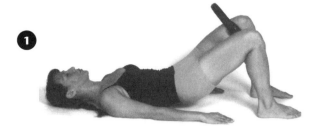

1

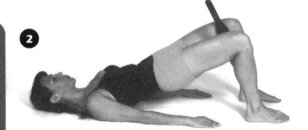

2

STARTING POSITION: Lie on your back, knees bent, feet flat on the floor, hip distance apart, with the circle or small ball between your knees. Door Frame arms are down by your sides, palms facing down. **INHALE TO BEGIN**.

1 EXHALE: Pull the navel to the spine and slowly roll your coccyx up off the mat, one vertebra at a time, until you come to the Bridge position. Make sure your hips are high enough so that your body makes one long line from shoulders to knees. Hold for one full breath.

2 INHALE, EXHALE, INHALE: Hold the Bridge.

EXHALE: Roll down one vertebra at a time, returning to starting position.

repeat **3 times**

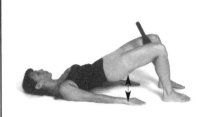

VARIATIONS

Bridge Pulses

Once up in the Bridge, gently pulse the hips up and down, squeezing the magic circle or small ball as you squeeze your glutes on every lift. Pulse 10 times, then hold the squeeze for 10 solid counts, then return to starting position. Repeat this sequence 3 times.

BENEFITS	DOS & DON'TS	IMAGINE
■ Teaches spinal articulation. ■ Strengthens the hamstrings and glutes.	■ Do keep your belly scooped in as you roll up to the Bridge. ■ Don't rise up so high that you hyper-extend your back. If you feel any back strain at all, lower the Bridge, scoop the belly in, and squeeze the glutes.	■ You are in the training scene from *Showgirls*.

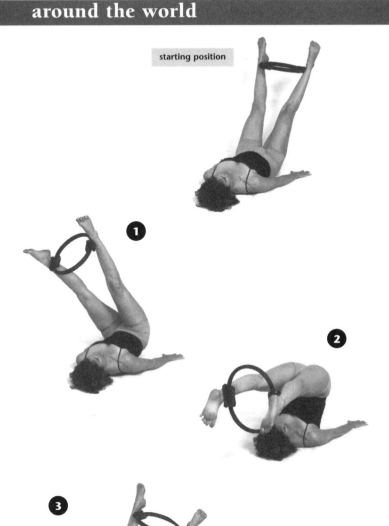

starting position

STARTING POSITION: Lie on your back with your legs up in a diagonal, the magic circle or small ball between your legs and Door Frame Arms down by your sides, palms facing down. Make sure to keep your belly pulled in and your low back flat on the floor. **INHALE TO BEGIN**.

1–2 **EXHALE**: Begin a large circle with your legs, lifting your hips up and to the left, then up and over your head.

3 Continue the circle, coming down toward your right, until you finish the circle in the starting position.

INHALE and reverse directions.

repeat 4 times

BENEFITS	DOS & DON'TS
■ Stretches and articulates the spine. ■ Strengthens the hip flexors, inner thighs, and abdominals, especially the obliques.	■ Don't roll onto your neck. ■ Keep pulling navel to spine. ■ Press Door Frame Arms onto the floor to help stabilize you.

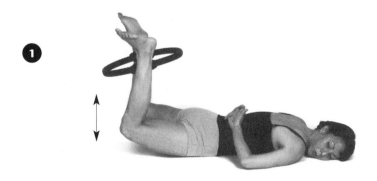

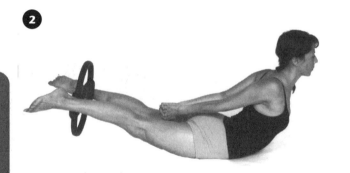

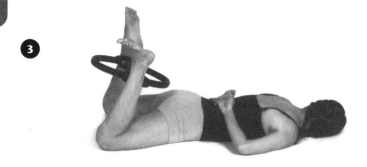

STARTING POSITION: Lie with your head to one side, your knees bent 90 degrees and the magic circle or small ball between your ankles. Your fingers should be interlaced behind you, with your elbows bent as much as possible and relaxed by your sides. **INHALE TO BEGIN**.

1 Squeeze your ankles together as you pulse the circle up to the sky three times.

2 EXHALE: Keep the thighs lifted up off the floor as you extend your legs behind you, straightening your arms back to lift your head and upper body off the floor, stretching your chest open.

3 INHALE: Return to the floor, with your head facing the opposite way, knees and arms bent in the starting position.

repeat **4 times**

BENEFITS	DOS & DON'TS
▪ Strengthens the butt, hamstrings, inner thighs, back, and neck extensors. ▪ Stretches the chest and belly.	▪ To avoid low back compression and maximize butt work, don't let your back arch when doing the pulses; instead, keep your pelvis tucked under, pressing your pubic bone down and lifting your belly up off the floor.

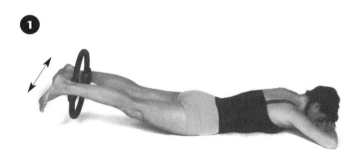

❶

STARTING POSITION: Lie on your belly, hands beneath your forehead, legs extended and externally rotated, with the magic circle between your heels, feet flexed.

1 INHALE AND EXHALE CONTINUOUSLY: Keep your belly scooped up off the mat and squeeze the circle in an even rhythm, controlling the in and the out movements, making a pulsing action. Alternate 10 pulses with feet flexed, 10 pulses feet pointed.

repeat **10 times**

circle/small ball

VARIATIONS

Up and Down

Keep the pulsing rhythm as you gradually lift the legs up on 4 pulses, and down on 4 pulses. Try pointing your feet for 8 counts, then flexing for 8. Repeat 4 sets of 8.

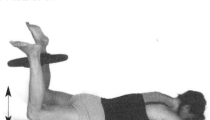

Bent Knee

Keep the circle between your ankles and bend the knees so the soles of the feet are facing the sky. Pull the navel up off the mat and press the pubic bone down onto the mat as you squeeze the circle, ever so slightly lifting the heels toward the sky as you squeeze. Repeat 10 times slowly.

Bent Knee to Straight

After the Bent Knee version, try extending the legs after each squeeze, only to bend them again. Squeeze, extend, bend, squeeze, extend, bend, etc., 10 more times.

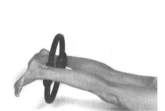
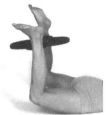

BENEFITS	DOS & DON'TS	IMAGINE
■ Strengthens and tones the butt and back of the thighs.	■ Don't hyperextend your lower back—instead, try to keep your belly scooped up off the mat and your pelvis tucked under.	■ You are firming your butt for bikini season.

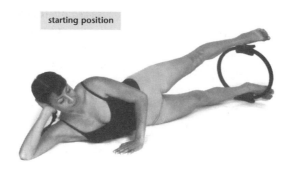

starting position

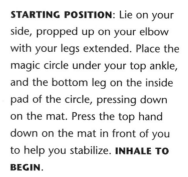

STARTING POSITION: Lie on your side, propped up on your elbow with your legs extended. Place the magic circle under your top ankle, and the bottom leg on the inside pad of the circle, pressing down on the mat. Press the top hand down on the mat in front of you to help you stabilize. **INHALE TO BEGIN**.

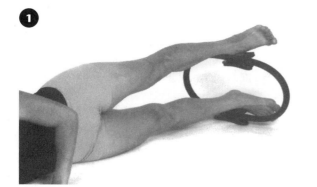

①

1–2 **EXHALE:** Pull the navel to the spine as you press the circle down. Control the circle back up.

repeat	10 times each side

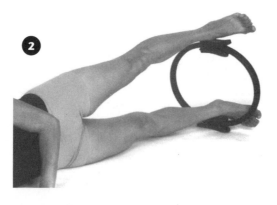

②

BENEFITS	DOS & DON'TS	IMAGINE
■ Strengthens the inner thighs. ■ Teaches the deep abdominal scoop and the synergistic connection between the oblique abdominals and the inner thighs.	■ Do release the circle on the inhale…give those inner thighs a rest! ■ Keep neutral spine when scooping and squeezing; its easy to tuck under during this part.	■ Your legs originate from your belly.

side lying series
bottom-leg pulse-ups
beginning

127

starting position

1

2

STARTING POSITION: Lie on your side, propped up on your elbow with your legs extended. Place the magic circle under your top ankle, and the bottom leg on the inside pad of the circle, pressing down on the mat. Press the top hand down on the mat in front of you to help you stabilize. **INHALE TO BEGIN.**

INHALE AND EXHALE CONTINUOUSLY: Keeping your belly scooped in, lift your bottom leg up to the top of the circle 10 times slowly. Then start with the lower leg up against the circle and pulse quickly up and down, accenting the "up" movement 10 times.

repeat **10 times each side**

circle/small ball

MODIFICATION

If your neck is strained in the propped up position, lower your head to the floor atop an extended lower arm.

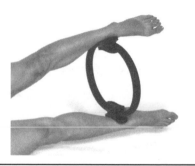

VARIATION

Put the magic circle between both ankles and lift it off the floor slightly, then squeeze the circle with both legs, pulsing in and out 10 times.

Try lifting the circle up as high as you can, then down. Repeat 10 times.

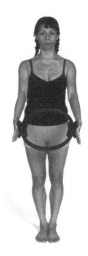

starting position

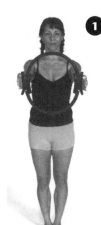

1

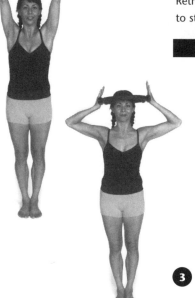

2

3

STARTING POSITION: From standing, hold the pads on either side of the magic circle out in front of you, arms extended low in front of your thighs. Stand in parallel, inner thighs squeezing together.

1–2 **INHALE AND EXHALE CONTINUOUSLY**: Squeeze the circle in an even rhythm, controlling both the in and the out movements. Every 4 squeezes, move the circle up—first straight in front of you, then above your head.

3 Pull the circle down by your ears, keeping your elbows wide and shoulders down. Retrograde the pulses back to starting position.

repeat **10 times**

BENEFITS	DOS & DON'TS	IMAGINE
▪ Strengthens the pecs.	▪ Do keep your belly scooped in. ▪ Do control the motion of the circle, especially on the "out" direction.	▪ We must, we must, we must improve our bust!

starting position

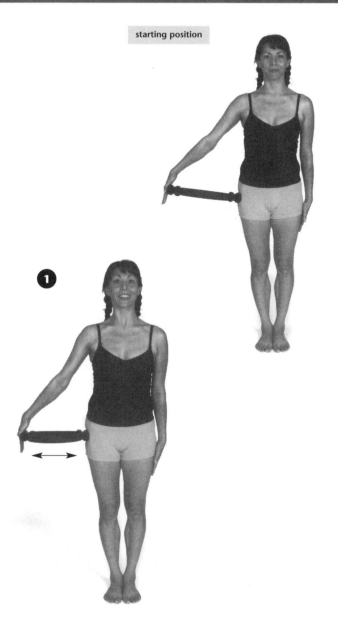

1

STARTING POSITION: Stand in parallel, inner thighs squeezing together. Hold the magic circle on your hip with one hand.

1 INHALE AND EXHALE CONTINUOUSLY: Squeeze the circle in an even rhythm, controlling both the in and the out movements.

repeat | 10 times

BENEFITS	DOS & DON'TS	IMAGINE
■ Strengthens the lats and pecs.	■ Do control the motion of the circle, especially on the "out" direction. ■ Do keep your belly scooped in.	■ You are holding a baby on your hip with all the right muscles!

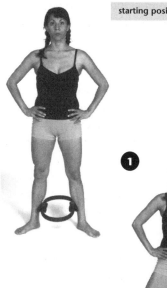

starting position

STARTING POSITION: Stand with the magic circle between your ankles, legs turned out from the tops of the hips. **INHALE TO BEGIN**.

1 **EXHALE**: Bend your knees, keeping your knees aligned over your second and third toes.

2 **INHALE**: Straighten your legs.

3 **EXHALE**: Rise onto your toes, keeping your knees aligned over your second and third toes. Return to starting position.

repeat **4 times**

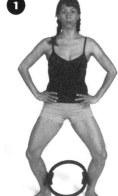

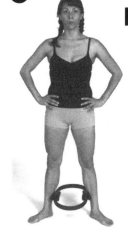

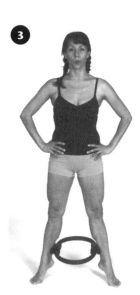

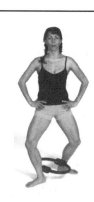

VARIATION

Fourth Position Plie

Stand in fourth position, one leg in front of the other, with the magic circle between your ankles. Then switch and do the other leg in front.

BENEFITS	DOS & DON'TS	IMAGINE
■ Strengthens the inner thighs. ■ Teaches balance and coordination.	■ Do keep your body aligned by scooping the belly in and keeping the shoulders relaxed down the back.	■ You are a ballet dancer doing your plie warm-up.

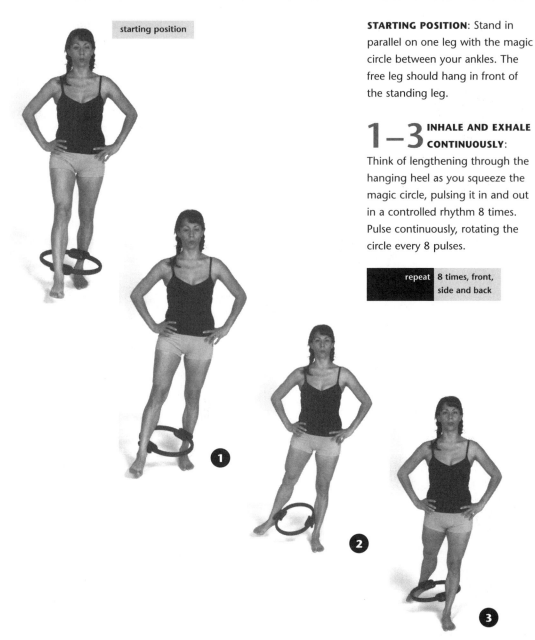

starting position

STARTING POSITION: Stand in parallel on one leg with the magic circle between your ankles. The free leg should hang in front of the standing leg.

1–3 INHALE AND EXHALE CONTINUOUSLY:

Think of lengthening through the hanging heel as you squeeze the magic circle, pulsing it in and out in a controlled rhythm 8 times. Pulse continuously, rotating the circle every 8 pulses.

repeat	8 times, front, side and back

circle/small ball

BENEFITS	DOS & DON'TS	IMAGINE
■ Strengthens the inner thighs. ■ Teaches balance and coordination.	■ Do use a wall to help balance if needed. ■ Do allow the hanging leg to really drop and lengthen out of the hip socket.	■ You are a pillar of stability.

STARTING POSITION: Stand in parallel on one leg with one foot atop the magic circle and arms crossed in "I Dream of Jeannie" position. **INHALE TO BEGIN**.

1 **EXHALE:** Slowly press the circle down.

INHALE and control back up to starting position.

repeat	8 times each side

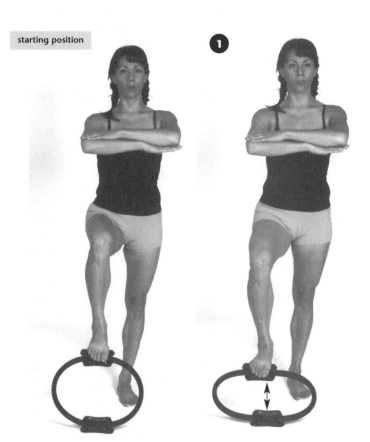

starting position

1

BENEFITS	DOS & DON'TS	IMAGINE
■ Teaches balance and coordination. ■ Good for knee/ankle instability.	■ Don't lock the standing knee—keep it soft.	■ This is harder than it looks.

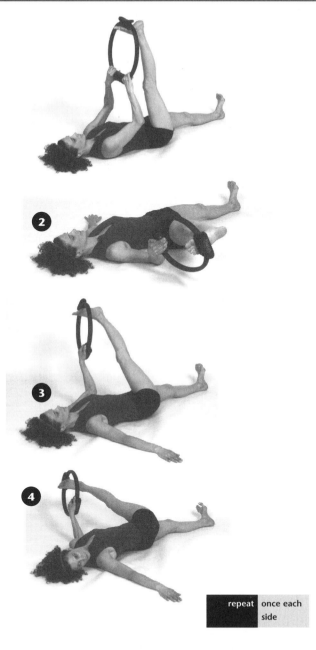

STARTING POSITION: Lie on your back, holding the magic circle, and place one foot inside the circle. Reach the leg up to the sky. **INHALE AND EXHALE CONTINUOUSLY**.

1 *Hamstring:* Reach the circle up to the sky, keeping the free leg either straight along the floor or, if you are very tight in your hamstrings, the knee bent and the foot placed on the floor. Keep your shoulders pulling down away from your ears, using your biceps to pull the circle closer to you. Use your quadriceps to straighten the leg. To increase the stretch, press your tailbone down onto the mat.

2 *Adductor:* From the Hamstring Stretch, hold the circle with the same hand as the foot in the circle and pull the circle to the side, allowing the hips to externally rotate. To increase the stretch, press your tailbone down onto the mat.

3 *Abductor:* From the Adductor Stretch, pull the magic circle back up to the sky, switch hands on the circle, then internally rotate the leg that is up in the air and slowly allow the leg to cross over the body. You don't have to go very far to feel this stretch on the outside of the leg and hip. To increase the stretch, press your tailbone down onto the mat.

4 *Spine Twist:* Keep reaching the leg across your body as far as you can, allowing your tailbone to come off the floor, feeling the belly scoop and the spine stretch; ground your free arm to the floor, trying to keep the shoulder blade pulling back to the floor.

repeat | once each side

BENEFITS	DOS & DON'TS	IMAGINE
■ Stretches the hip muscles.	■ Don't allow tension to come into the neck and shoulders; keep the shoulders down away from the ears and use your biceps to help you pull the circle for a deeper stretch.	■ You will have open hips someday.

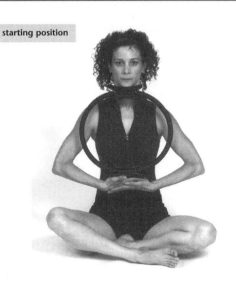

starting position

STARTING POSITION: Sit cross-legged or on a chair, holding the magic circle under your chin with the pad touching the chin. **INHALE TO BEGIN**.

1 EXHALE: Press the circle down with your chin, thinking about lengthening the back of the neck.

INHALE and control back up to the starting position.

repeat **8 times**

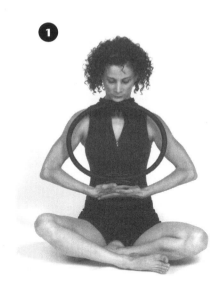

1

BENEFITS	DOS & DON'TS	IMAGINE
■ Strengthens the neck flexors. ■ Can help correct forward head posture. ■ Gives traction to the neck.	■ Don't jut your chin forward when pressing; instead, keep the circle close to the body. ■ Do go slowly and control the movement, especially in the return phase.	■ This actually feels good.

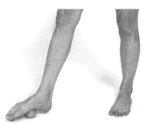

starting position

STARTING POSITION: First, roll out your feet with the pinkie ball (see page 136). Then sit on a chair with feet hip distance apart, legs in parallel, with the small ball (or magic circle) between your knees.

1–2 **INHALE TO BEGIN**: Sit up tall. **EXHALE**: Squeeze the small ball with your inner thighs while simultaneously lifting up the inner arches of your feet. Think "short foot," meaning you are making your feet a little shorter by lifting up the arches. Repeat 5 times.

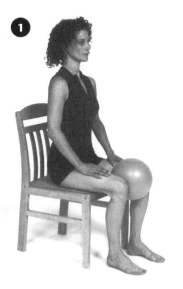

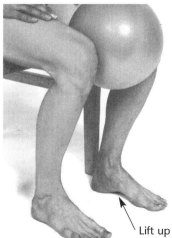

3 Remove the small ball and stand up on your feet without moving them, feeling your arch/inner thigh connection while standing.

repeat **8 times**

 Lift up the arch, thus "shortening the foot."

circle/small ball

BENEFITS	DOS & DON'TS	IMAGINE
■ Increases the arch of the foot. ■ Strengthens the intrinsic muscles of the foot.	■ To help find your arch/inner thigh connection, "flick" the muscles on by flicking your fingers along the line from your arches to the inner thighs with quick light movements. This gives the brain a more concrete connection. ■ Do keep pressing the metatarsals (balls of your feet) down onto the floor, especially pressing the big toe metatarsals. ■ Do keep the toes relaxed as much as possible and try to do the exercise from the intrinsic foot muscles, not the toes.	■ There is line of energy connecting your arch with your inner thigh, as if there is a string originating from your arch that follows along the inner leg up to the inner thigh. When you squeeze the circle, you are pulling the arch up with it.

muscle releases

starting position

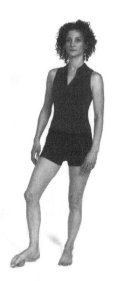

STARTING POSITION: Stand up with one foot on the pinkie ball.

INHALE AND EXHALE CONTINU-OUSLY: Roll out the bottom of your foot, applying as much pressure as you can stand. Try rolling up and down the foot as well as side to side.

repeat	until released

pinkie ball

1

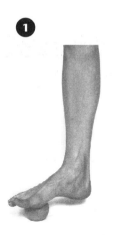

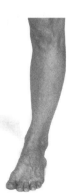

2

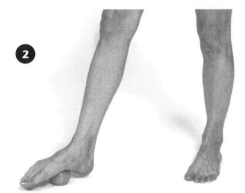

BENEFITS	DOS & DON'TS	IMAGINE
■ Releases the fascia of the foot. ■ Can help relieve foot and heel pain and increase articulation of the foot.	■ Do focus on the arch area. ■ Do this before doing Short Foot (page 135).	■ You are rolling out years of foot tension.

glutes and rotators release *beginning*

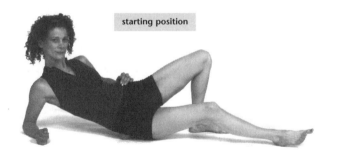

starting position

STARTING POSITION: Sit on the side of your hip, with the pinkie ball under the side of your butt. Roll back and forth, up and down, focusing on tight areas.

repeat	until released

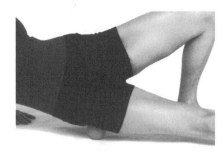

TFL release *beginning*

starting position

STARTING POSITION: Lie on your side, propped up on one elbow. Put the pinkie ball in the side/front crease of your hip, where the thigh bone meets the hip bone. Allow your weight to drop into the ball and try some micromovements to find the tightest fibers.

repeat	until released

1

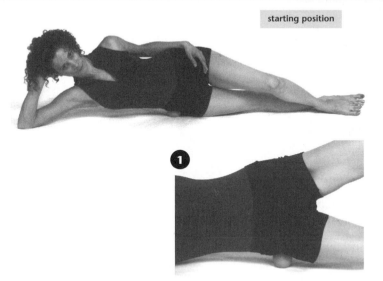

pinkie ball

BENEFITS	DOS & DON'TS	IMAGINE
■ *Glutes and Rotators Release:* Releases your glutes and external rotators. ■ *TFL Release:* Releases the TFL, which can help free the hips and may help alleviate hip pain.	■ Do bring your awareness to exactly where you are tight and focus on those places. ■ Do breathe into the release.	■ *Glutes and Rotators Release:* Your butt can be free of tension. ■ *TFL Release:* Your leg is getting longer with every exhale.

starting position

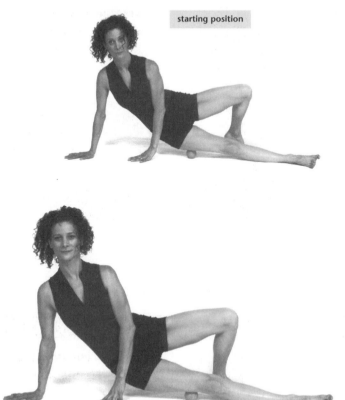

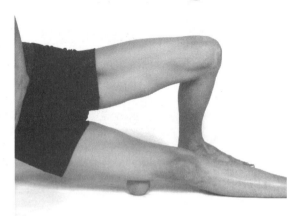

STARTING POSITION: Sit on the side of your hip with the pinkie ball under the lateral side of your bottom thigh. Use your arms to support your weight, and allow the top leg to bend. Place the foot on the mat to help you balance.

INHALE AND EXHALE CONTINU-OUSLY: Roll slowly up and down the lateral side of your lower leg, releasing the IT band that runs from the side of your knee all the way up to the side of your hip. This will be painful, especially where there is tightness, so focus on those painful areas.

| repeat | until released |

pinkie ball

BENEFITS	DOS & DON'TS	IMAGINE
■ Releases the IT band. ■ Can help with lateral knee pain, hip pain, and back pain.	■ Don't roll over your knee. ■ Breathe through the pain. ■ Don't continue if you notice knee instability afterward.	■ The endorphins will put you in a good mood.

pec release   *beginning*

starting position

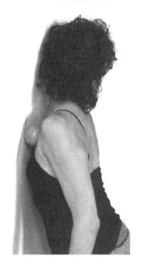

STARTING POSITION: Stand facing a wall with the front of your armpit pressed into the pinkie ball.

INHALE AND EXHALE CONTINU-OUSLY: Press as much weight as you can stand into the ball and roll your body up and down and back and forth, massaging out the pectoral muscles.

repeat	30–60 seconds each side

trap release   *beginning*

starting position

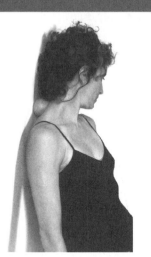

STARTING POSITION: Stand with your back to the wall and the pinkie ball placed at the top of your shoulder.

INHALE AND EXHALE CONTINU-OUSLY: Roll back and forth and up and down on the upper trapezius muscle (where the neck meets the shoulders). Focus on any particularly tight or knotty areas.

repeat	30–60 seconds each side

pinkie ball

BENEFITS	DOS & DON'TS	IMAGINE
■ *Pec Release:* Releases the pecs. ■ *Trap Release:* Releases the upper trapezius muscle.	■ Do get in there with the ball. ■ Do lean into the wall and adjust body position to get the "trigger" point on the top of the shoulder.	■ *Pec Release:* You are getting intimate with the wall. ■ *Trap Release:* You can release all that computer tension.

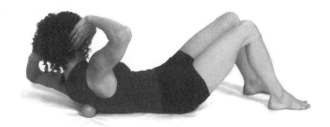

starting position

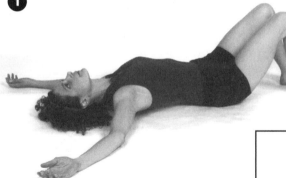

1

STARTING POSITION: Lie on your back on the mat with the pinkie ball wherever you feel a knot in your upper back.

INHALE AND EXHALE CONTINUOUSLY: Press your weight into the ball and roll around until you find your knot. Then focus on releasing this area by rolling back and forth and up and down. To increase the pressure, lift up your hips.

1 You can also increase the pressure by lying back on the ball and rolling back and forth, making micromovements.

repeat	30–60 seconds each knot

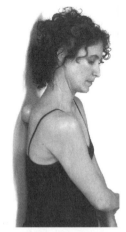

VARIATION

This release can also be done standing with your back to the wall and the pinkie ball wherever you feel a knot in your upper back. Roll around until you find your knot and then focus on releasing this area by rolling back and forth and up and down the wall.

BENEFITS	DOS & DON'TS	IMAGINE
■ Releases spot tension in the upper back.	■ Do experiment with different angles to get the best release.	■ You can find that trouble spot and let it go!

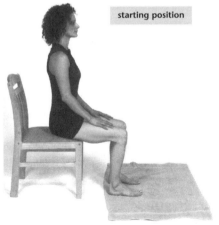

starting position

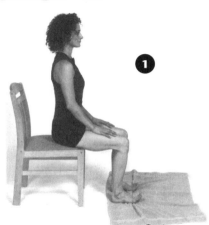

1

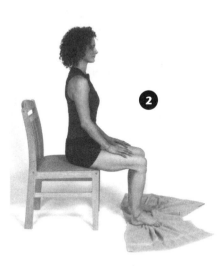

2

STARTING POSITION: Sit on a chair with a towel on the floor under your feet.

1–2 INHALE AND EXHALE CONTINUOUSLY:

Keeping your heels on the floor, lift the balls of your feet and pull the towel toward your heels, pressing your metatarsals into the towel and lifting up the arches of the feet as you do so. Once you have reached the top of the towel, reverse the motion and press the towel back to starting position.

repeat once

BENEFITS	DOS & DON'TS	IMAGINE
■ Increases the arch of the foot. ■ Strengthens the intrinsic muscles of the foot.	■ Don't pull with the toes; instead, pull with the ball of your foot. ■ Do keep the big toe metatarsals pressing into the floor to ensure you are maximizing the intrinsic muscles of the feet rather than the toe muscles.	■ You are shortening the foot as you pull the towel in.

index

Prop abbreviations used in index: EB (exercise band), MC (magic circle), PB (pinkie ball), R (roller), SB (small ball), and T (towel).

other books by ulysses press

ELLIE HERMAN'S PILATES WORKBOOK ON THE BALL: ILLUSTRATED STEP-BY-STEP GUIDE
Ellie Herman, $13.95
Combines the powerful slimming and shaping effects of Pilates with the low-impact, high-intensity workout of the ball.

PILATES WORKBOOK: ILLUSTRATED STEP-BY-STEP GUIDE TO MATWORK TECHNIQUES
Michael King, $12.95
Illustrates the core matwork movements exactly as Joseph Pilates intended them to be performed; readers learn each movement by following the photographic sequences and explanatory captions.

WEIGHTS ON THE BALL WORKBOOK: STEP-BY-STEP GUIDE WITH OVER 350 PHOTOS
Steven Stiefel, $14.95
With exercises suited for all skill levels, *Weights on the Ball Workbook* shows how to simultaneously use weights and the exercise ball for the ultimate total-body workout.

YOGA THERAPIES: 45 SEQUENCES TO RELIEVE STRESS, DEPRESSION, REPETITIVE STRAIN, SPORTS INJURIES AND MORE
Jessie Chapman   photographs by Dhyan, $14.95
Featuring an artistic presentation, this book is filled with beautifully photographed sequences that relieve stress, release anger, relax back muscles and reverse repetitive strain injuries.

To order these books call 800-377-2542 or 510-601-8301, fax 510-601-8307, e-mail ulysses@ulyssespress.com, or write to Ulysses Press, P.O. Box 3440, Berkeley, CA 94703. All retail orders are shipped free of charge. California residents must include sales tax. Allow two to three weeks for delivery.